THE ART OF DESIGNING PERFUME

A PRACTICAL GUIDE TO NATURAL PERFUME DESIGN

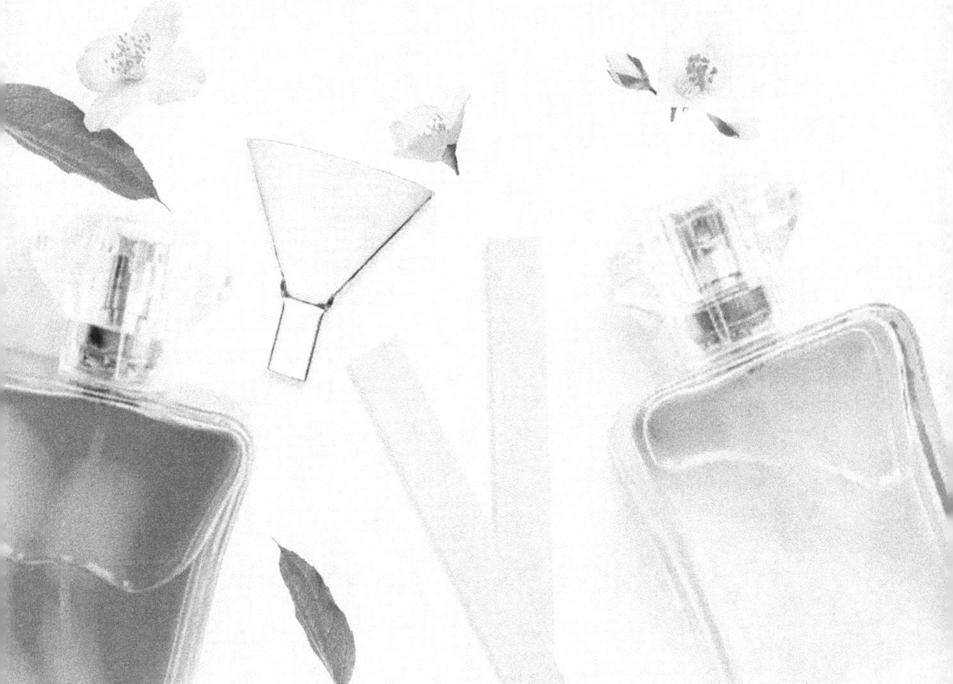

REBECCA PARK TOTILO

The Art of Designing Perfume:
A Practical Guide to Natural Perfume Design

The Natural Perfume Series — Book Two

Printed in the United States of America.

Published by Rebecca at the Well Foundation.

Paperback ISBN: 979-8-9937841-0-6
Electronic ISBN: 979-8-9937841-2-0

Contents

Introduction to Designing Perfume with Structure and Intention

Fragrance is often spoken of as art—an expression of beauty, emotion, or personal sensibility. While this is true, it is only part of the story. A perfume is also an orchestrated experience, shaped by proportion, timing, and the quiet influence of repetition. Its impact lies not merely in what is chosen, but in how it is composed.

Materials are selected not only for their scent, but for their behavior—how they rise, diffuse, soften, and linger. Structure determines whether a fragrance feels effortless or unsettled, radiant or restrained. Endurance arises from harmony rather than force, refinement rather than excess, and intention rather than novelty.

This book approaches perfumery not as an elusive art, but as a disciplined craft practiced with clarity and discernment. It is written for perfumers who wish to compose with deliberation—to translate vision into form, to shape accords with precision, to guide aromatic evolution with quiet control.

Natural materials are uniquely suited to this philosophy. Botanical essences unfold in measured stages, allowing perfume to be composed as a progression: an opening that invites, a heart that sustains, a foundation that settles with grace.

Throughout these pages, fragrance is treated as a living system rather than a collection of notes. The examples are not meant to be copied, but to demonstrate principle. The aim is not imitation but understanding—so that each fragrance may reflect both mastery and personal voice.

A well-composed perfume does not announce itself. It reveals itself through its unfolding, its restraint, and its presence over time.

How to Read This Book

As you move through these pages, hold one central question in mind:

What experience is this fragrance intended to create, and how does its composition support that intention?

This book can be read in sequence, but it does not require a rigid order. Readers may enter at different points, depending on their experience and purpose.

For those new to structural design, Chapters 1–5 establish shared language and foundational principles. These chapters examine how fragrance is perceived, how compositional structure shapes that perception, and how materials function within an aromatic framework.

If your focus is blending and formulation, Chapters 11–14 guide you from concept to finished concentrate, addressing technique, accord development, and deliberate formulation methods.

For refinement and critical evaluation, Chapter 17 explores assessment and iteration, while Chapter 21 offers solutions to common formulation challenges. Chapter 15 expands into advanced structural development, and Chapter 19 examines adaptation across product formats. Chapter 20 brings these elements together in a complete design sequence, guiding you through conceptualizing, building, diluting, and evaluating a perfume as a cohesive act of structured creation.

The examples show how structure works in practice, supporting confident, informed design.

CHAPTER 1
Where Design Meets Sensory Experience

Fragrance exists at the intersection of perception and structure. While it is often described in emotional terms—uplifting, comforting, seductive—its effects arise from deliberate choices: material selection, proportion, volatility, and timing. Scent is not passive. It is received, interpreted, and remembered through repetition and context.

This chapter establishes the foundation for intentional perfume design. Fragrance is not mere decoration or intuition. It is an orchestrated sensory experience shaped by proportion, progression, and material behavior. A perfume's effectiveness lies not in what it claims, but in how it unfolds and endures over time.

Fragrance as Designed Sensory Input

Every perfume delivers information to the senses. From the first moment of contact, scent signals intensity, direction, familiarity, and change. These signals influence attention and perception before conscious interpretation occurs. Whether a fragrance feels bright or heavy, fleeting or persistent, stimulating or settling is the result of structure.

Structured perfume design begins by asking:

- How does this perfume enter awareness?
- How does it evolve as it develops?
- What kind of presence does it maintain?
- How does it resolve?

These questions shift perfume-making away from ingredient–driven choices and toward experience–based design. Materials are selected not only for how they smell, but for the role they play within the structure.

Why Natural Perfume Is Especially Suited to Functional Design

Natural perfume materials are inherently dynamic. Essential oils and botanical extracts contain complex aromatic profiles that unfold gradually, never static. This evolution makes natural fragrance especially responsive to time, temperature, and skin chemistry.

Because natural perfumes change, they can be composed as sequences instead of fixed impressions. A fragrance may open with clarity and lift, settle into a sustained center, and resolve into a grounded finish. Each phase contributes to the overall experience.

Intentional structure is designed to support the materials' natural progression. Instead of forcing uniformity, the perfumer guides progression—allowing materials to express themselves while maintaining coherence through proportion, balance, and timing. This approach values observation, patience, and restraint over rigid control.

Structure as the Foundation of Function

Structure is the underlying framework that determines whether a fragrance feels clear or confused, balanced or fatiguing. Without cohesion, even beautiful materials can leave an indistinct impression. With thoughtful arrangement, relatively simple formulas can feel complete and deliberate.

Composition governs the pacing of evaporation, the relationship between top, heart, and base, the clarity of transitions, and the balance between projection and intimacy.

A fragrance intended for frequent daytime wear may prioritize lightness and transparency, while one suited to evening or personal ritual may emphasize continuity and depth. These distinctions arise from compositional decisions, not ornamentation.

Throughout this book, structure is treated as a primary skill. You will learn how to create perfumes that perform consistently through extended wear, guided by proportion, balance, and timing.

Fragrance, Repetition, and Context

One of the defining characteristics of perfume design is its relationship to repetition. A scent worn once is simply perceived. A scent worn consistently within the same context becomes familiar and associated.

When fragrance is paired repeatedly with an activity—work, rest, reflection, or transition—it begins to align with that experience through sensory memory. This association does not require explanation or intention; it develops naturally through repeated use and context.

For the perfumer, this means considering not only how a fragrance smells, but when and how it will be worn. A perfume intended for daily focus must remain comfortable and clear over repeated wear. A fragrance created for evening or personal ritual must settle and sustain rather than demand attention. These considerations influence material selection, proportion, and overall structure.

The Role of the Perfumer as Designer

In professional perfumery, the perfumer acts as a composer. This work requires intention, evaluation, and refinement. Decisions are guided by how a fragrance performs across stages of evaporation, not by novelty or accumulation.

This discipline does not diminish creativity—it sharpens it. When the perfumer understands how materials behave within a structure, creative choices become precise and confident instead of abstract and uncertain.

Throughout this book, you'll learn to observe before adjusting, subtract before adding, and evaluate a fragrance as it develops. You'll design perfumes to be worn and experienced—not simply displayed. These principles support disciplined practice, whether you create for personal use, teaching, or product development.

Moving Forward

Designing perfume with structure is a disciplined way of working. It values clarity, intention, and experience over excess or ornamentation, and approaches scent deliberately rather than assuming it.

The chapters that follow develop the skills required to work at this level. You will train the nose, build and evaluate accords, understand how composition influences perception, and apply professional methods to natural perfumery.

By the end of this book, you will not only know how to make perfume—you will understand why it succeeds when it succeeds, and how to create fragrances that perform consistently over successive evaluations.

Chapter 2

From Tradition to Modern Perfumery

Modern perfumery did not emerge in isolation. Many of the perfume formats, concentration types, and application styles used today evolved from earlier cultural and practical traditions. Understanding these origins provides context for why perfumes are structured, diluted, and applied as they are, particularly when working with natural materials.

Here we don't present perfume history for its own sake. Instead, it uses selected historical and cultural references to explain how perfume types and concentration standards developed and why certain formats remain relevant in natural perfumery. The focus is functional orientation: how perfumes are categorized, applied, and experienced, and how those choices influence structure, longevity, and use.

Perfume by Concentration

Perfumes are categorized by the strength of their aromatic compounds diluted in alcohol or a carrier oil. Higher concentrations generally result in greater intensity and longer-lasting fragrance.

Modern concentration categories such as parfum, eau de parfum, and eau de toilette evolved from traditional strength classifications and remain relevant in contemporary natural perfumery. Detailed dilution ranges and professional application standards are covered in Chapter 9.

In natural perfumery, these classifications still apply, though the solvent is often a carrier oil such as jojoba or fractionated coconut oil instead of alcohol. This alters wear characteristics, typically resulting in softer diffusion and closer skin presence compared to alcohol-based perfumes.

Perfume types can also be defined by how they are applied. Traditional alcohol-based sprays are the most familiar, especially in fine fragrance. However, natural perfumery allows for a range of more hands-on application formats. Perfume oils, for instance, are essential oil blends diluted in a fixed oil and applied directly to pulse points. These offer a more intimate scent experience with less projection. Roll-on perfumes are a convenient format for on-the-go application, while solid perfumes—made with a base of beeswax and oil—are well-suited for travel and provide a concentrated, long-lasting scent.

Some prefer hydrosol–based mists, which combine essential oils with aromatic waters or alcohol to create lightweight body or room sprays. These are particularly useful for seasonal blends, facial mists, or refreshing daytime scents. Each application method produces a different wear profile and serves a distinct role within a perfumer's range of formats.

Another way perfumes have traditionally been categorized is by gender designation, although this is increasingly becoming obsolete. Historically, floral and powdery perfumes were marketed as feminine, while woody, spicy, or musky scents were labeled masculine. Citrus and herbal fragrances often fell into a more neutral or "unisex" category. In natural perfumery, where personalization is emphasized and ingredients are chosen for their functional roles, divisions tend to fade. Scents are selected to resonate with mood, intention, or personality rather than gender norms.

Finally, perfumes may also be identified by cultural or historical tradition. For example, attars are alcohol–free perfumes developed in India and the Middle East, where botanicals are distilled directly into sandalwood or other base oils. These are highly concentrated and deeply aromatic. In 18th–century Europe, eau de cologne became popular as a refreshing, citrus–based formulation intended for daily hygiene and revitalization. Pomanders and sachets, used in medieval and Renaissance Europe, were solid or pouch–based scent carriers kept in garments or worn as accessories. Ancient Egypt developed its own signature style with kyphi—a rich, resinous blend of herbs, spices, and honey, burned as incense or worn in wax cones during rituals.

These traditional types still inspire modern perfumers, who draw on history, ritual, and cultural storytelling to craft scents deeply rooted in both place and purpose.

Perfume Types by Traditional Gender Category

Although natural perfumery increasingly resists rigid gender classifications, traditional perfumery has historically grouped scents into broad marketing categories. "Masculine" fragrances were typically built around earthy, woody, fougère, or spicy materials such as vetiver, cedarwood, and patchouli, while "feminine" perfumes often emphasized floral, sweet, or powdery compositions featuring materials like rose, ylang ylang, and jasmine. "Unisex" fragrances tended to balance fresh, citrus, or herbal elements—such as bergamot, lavender, or frankincense—designed to appeal across the gender spectrum rather than conform to a single identity.

Modern perfumery increasingly recognizes scent as a personal experience, not a gendered one.

CHAPTER 3
The Structure of a Fragrance

Structural Timing in Perfume Design

In perfume design, top, heart, and base are best understood as timing functions as opposed to rigid categories. Each stage reveals which elements are meant to lead at a given moment and how the fragrance transitions from one phase to the next. Structural timing allows the designer to anticipate change instead of reacting to it.

The opening establishes the initial impression and diffusion. It is often defined by volatile or high–impact elements that create lift and clarity, but it must be carefully supported to avoid rapid collapse. The heart defines the fragrance's identity—the stage where balance is most critical and where the design intention should be most clearly expressed. The base provides continuity, depth, and persistence, anchoring the fragrance and carrying it through extended wear.

Effective structure depends on designing when dominance shifts, not simply what materials are present. This timing informs proportion, layering decisions, and the placement of supporting elements so the fragrance remains cohesive as it evolves.

Balance as a Design Principle

In perfume design, balance is measured by behavior, not by fixed ratios. A fragrance is balanced when it develops smoothly over time—without abrupt gaps, excessive heaviness, or loss of identity as it moves from opening to drydown. Imbalance reveals itself through performance, not numbers.

A weak opening often indicates insufficient lift or poor transition into the heart. A hollow or fleeting heart suggests inadequate structural support. An overly dense or muddy drydown typically points to base elements that overpower instead of stabilizing the composition. These issues are not resolved by mechanically adjusting formulas, but by revisiting structure—reconsidering proportion, timing, and functional placement.

Balanced perfume design is confirmed through repeated observation. The fragrance is evaluated at intervals, and adjustments are made based on its behavior at each stage of wear. The goal is continuity, clarity, and alignment with the original design intention—not adherence to predetermined blending rules.

Understanding structure clarifies *what a fragrance needs to do* before any materials are selected. Once timing, balance, and functional roles are defined, materials can be chosen with purpose rather than solely through experimentation. The next chapter shifts attention to essential oils—not as ingredients to combine, but as design tools whose behavior, strengths, and limitations determine how structure is executed in practice.

16

CHAPTER 4

Essential Oils as Perfume Materials

Essential oils form the foundation of natural perfumery. These concentrated aromatic extracts are obtained from plants through physical processes such as steam distillation, cold pressing, or carbon dioxide extraction. Each essential oil contains a complex profile of aromatic constituents that shape its scent, diffusion, and longevity.

Unlike synthetic fragrance materials, essential oils are inherently variable. Botanical species, growing conditions, harvest timing, and extraction method all influence aroma. Lavender grown at high altitude may smell noticeably different from lavender grown at sea level, and oils distilled from the same plant at different times of year can vary in both scent and behavior. This natural variability gives botanical perfumes their depth and individuality.

Essential oils behave dynamically on the skin, evolving as lighter components evaporate and heavier molecules emerge. This progression creates the layered experience characteristic of natural perfume. Understanding how and when an oil reveals itself helps the perfumer determine its role within the fragrance.

In perfumery, essential oils are selected not only for their aroma but for the role they play within a structure. Some materials provide lift and brightness, others contribute to the heart's continuity, and still others anchor the composition and extend its presence. An oil that smells beautiful on its own may behave differently when blended, and learning to anticipate these shifts is part of developing aromatic skill.

Essential oils differ from synthetic fragrance materials in both composition and behavior. While synthetic materials are often engineered for uniformity and consistency, essential oils contain dozens of naturally occurring constituents that interact with each other. This complexity allows for nuance and depth, but it also requires patience and restraint. Natural perfumery rewards thoughtful blending and careful evaluation over time.

Working with essential oils requires a responsive, observant approach to perfume design. The perfumer does not force materials into predetermined roles; instead, they evaluate how the materials behave—adjusting ratios, allowing blends to rest, and observing changes as they unfold. This process builds technical understanding and strengthens the ability to structure perfumes with clarity and control.

With an understanding of how essential oils behave individually, the next step is to learn how they interact within a structure.

CHAPTER 5
Fragrance Families as Design Frameworks

Fragrance families provide a shared language for understanding scent. They help perfumers organize aromatic materials, recognize patterns, and design fragrances with intention instead of guesswork. While scent perception is inherently subjective, fragrance families offer a practical framework for translating sensory impressions into structure.

At their core, fragrance families group materials according to dominant aromatic characteristics. These groupings are not rigid rules, but design tools that help anticipate how materials may interact and how a composition may be perceived as it unfolds. Many contemporary perfumes draw from multiple families, creating hybrid structures that feel complex while remaining coherent.

Understanding fragrance families supports every stage of perfume design—from material selection and blending to evaluation and refinement. They also provide a way to articulate design decisions clearly, whether working independently, teaching others, or formulating at a professional level.

The Four Primary Fragrance Families

Most perfumes are built around one or more of four primary fragrance families: **Floral, Woody, Fresh, and Amber** (often referred to as **Oriental**). These families provide a structural framework for understanding scent character and organizing materials within a composition.

Floral fragrances are centered on flower–derived aromas and often form the heart of a perfume. They can range from light and transparent to rich and opulent. A floral composition may feature a single dominant material or a blended bouquet of multiple florals. Common materials include rose, jasmine, neroli, ylang ylang, lavender, and geranium. Depending on structure and supporting notes, florals may feel soft, romantic, green, spicy, or creamy.

Woody fragrances draw their character from woods, roots, and resinous or earthy materials. These compositions tend to feel grounding, warm, and stable, often forming the structural base of a perfume. Cedarwood, sandalwood, vetiver, patchouli, and amyris are common woody materials. While woods frequently anchor a composition, they may also appear in the heart, shaping the fragrance's overall weight and continuity.

Fresh fragrances are defined by brightness, clarity, and immediacy. This family includes citrus, green, aromatic, and watery impressions. Citrus oils such as bergamot, lemon, grapefruit, and sweet orange are classic fresh materials and are commonly used as top notes. Green and aromatic materials—such as basil, rosemary, galbanum, and petitgrain—add crispness and lift. Fresh structures often require careful anchoring to maintain balance and persistence over time.

Amber (Oriental) fragrances are warm, resinous, and often sensual. They rely on balsams, resins, and sweet materials such as benzoin, labdanum, vanilla, frankincense, and myrrh. Amber fragrances provide richness and depth, often forming the foundation of evening or colder-weather perfumes. These materials also act as natural fixatives, helping to extend wear time.

Secondary and Hybrid Fragrance Families

Beyond primary families, several secondary families offer additional nuance and complexity.

Chypre fragrances combine freshness with depth, traditionally built around a contrast between citrus top notes and mossy, resinous bases. Bergamot, oakmoss, labdanum, and patchouli are classic components. Chypre perfumes feel elegant, structured, and sophisticated.

Fougère fragrances, meaning "fern-like," typically feature lavender, aromatic herbs, and a warm base. These perfumes feel clean and classic, often associated with barbershop-style compositions.

Gourmand fragrances suggest edible warmth and sweetness. In natural perfumery, gourmand effects are implied rather than literal, using materials like vanilla, benzoin, cocoa, tonka bean, and sweet citrus notes.

Green fragrances emphasize leafy, fresh–cut, or vegetal impres-sions. Materials such as galbanum, violet leaf, basil, and green mandarin contribute crispness and clarity.

Leather fragrances are smoky, rugged, and bold. In natural per-fumery, leather effects are created through accords using birch tar, cade, labdanum, and smoky resins, not animal–derived materials.

How Oils Shift Families by Proportion

An essential oil does not belong permanently to a single fra-grance family. Its role depends on how it is used within a compo-sition. For example, bergamot may function as a bright citrus top note in one perfume, or act as a unifying element bridging floral and woody structures in another. Patchouli can feel earthy and heavy at higher concentrations, or smooth and grounding when used in trace amounts.

Understanding how proportion shapes perception is essential. Small adjustments can shift a perfume's overall character—moving it from fresh to warm, or from floral to woody. This flexibility is part of what makes natural perfumery expressive and responsive.

Why Fragrance Families Matter in Design

Fragrance families provide structure without limiting creativity. They help you predict interactions, balance contrasting elements, and design perfumes that feel intentional not accidental. When you understand these categories, you gain greater confidence in both creating and evaluating fragrance.

As you continue through this book, fragrance families will serve as reference points instead of boundaries—guiding your choices while leaving room for personal interpretation.

CHAPTER 6
Training the Nose: Professional Olfactory Skills

Olfactory Training and Sensory Development

Training the nose is the deliberate development of olfactory perception and discrimination. This skill is foundational in perfume design, as it sharpens awareness of structure, nuance, and material behavior over time. With consistent, intentional practice, the nose learns to recognize individual notes, accords, and transitions within complex fragrances.

The focus here centralizes all instructions related to smelling, evaluating, and assessing aroma. While other chapters reference observation and adjustment, the methods for perceiving structure and making informed decisions are established here to ensure clarity and consistency throughout the book.

Start with Basic Scents

Begin with materials that are easily recognizable—citrus (lemon, orange), floral (rose, lavender), herbal (mint, basil), and woody (cedarwood, sandalwood). Work with single materials on blotters or in isolation to familiarize yourself with their core character before moving on to more complex compositions.

Build a Personal Scent Library

Develop a collection of essential oils, absolutes, and aroma materials representing a broad range of scent categories, including fruity, floral, spicy, woody, and resinous. Label and organize materials clearly so they are easy to access during evaluation and design work. Over time, this library becomes a critical professional reference.

Practice Scent Recognition

Regular exposure strengthens olfactory recognition. Blind smelling exercises—testing materials without looking at the label—sharpen perception and reduce assumptions. Scent memory exercises, where previously smelled materials are revisited and identified, reinforce long-term recognition and confidence.

Focus on Individual Notes

Train the nose to isolate individual notes within complex fragrances. As you smell, identify which materials contribute brightness, warmth, softness, or depth. Associating specific sensory characteristics with specific materials builds clarity and analytical confidence.

Use Comparative Analysis

Comparative smelling is one of the most effective professional tools. Smelling materials side by side reveals distinctions that are often missed when evaluated individually. For example, comparing Bulgarian rose and Damask rose highlights differences in sweetness, spice, and depth. Comparison refines discrimination and reduces vague or generalized impressions.

Develop a Sensory Vocabulary

Cultivate a consistent descriptive vocabulary that translates perception into usable language. Terms such as citrus, floral, spicy, resinous, earthy, herbaceous, and woody support clear analysis and communication. Personal associations may aid memory, but professional vocabulary ensures consistency.

Evaluate Progress Over Time

Track improvements in accuracy and confidence through regular documentation. Note challenges, shifts in perception, and materials that require further study. Self–evaluation supports continuous refinement and skill development.

Apply Skills in Context

Olfactory training supports every stage of perfume design—evaluating materials, assessing blends, identifying imbalance, and guiding structural decisions. Practical application reinforces learning and strengthens intuitive understanding of fragrance behavior.

Practice Patience and Consistency

Olfactory development is cumulative. Progress emerges through repeated exposure, attention, and time. Each session builds sensitivity, clarity, and confidence, forming a foundation that strengthens over an entire career.

Smelling with Intention

Casual or reflexive smelling is insufficient for professional perfumery. Intentional smelling requires attention, pacing, and repetition. Smelling directly from the bottle reveals only the most volatile components and provides an incomplete impression. Structured evaluation methods are essential to understand how a material behaves over time.

Using Perfume Blotters for Evaluation

Perfume blotters are the primary evaluation tool. Label the wider paddle end of the blotter and dip only the narrow tip into the material. Keep the blotter upright so the scented tip does not come into contact with the workspace.

As evaporation occurs, the aromatic life cycle becomes visible, allowing evaluation of the opening, heart, and drydown without interference from skin chemistry.

How to Smell Correctly

Hold the blotter approximately one inch from the nose and gently wave it instead of inhaling directly. After the first impression, pause to allow the brain to process sensory information. Smell again after a brief interval and observe changes in character, intensity, and texture. Structural perception develops through repeated observation over time.

Understanding Drydown and Structural Perception

Aromatic materials contain many molecules that evaporate at different rates. Initial impressions reflect top–note components, followed by heart notes and finally base notes as evaporation slows.

On blotters, top notes may be detectable for several days, heart notes for about a week, and base notes for weeks or longer. Observing this progression trains the nose to recognize structural roles and predict material behavior in finished perfumes.

Organoleptic Evaluation

Organoleptic evaluation assesses aromatic materials using the senses—primarily smell—along with visual and physical observation. While analytical testing provides chemical data, organoleptic evaluation reveals how a material performs in design.

Observe aroma clarity, evolution, color, viscosity, and texture. These factors provide insight into quality, age, and usability. Taste is traditionally included in organoleptic evaluation, but is neither required nor appropriate for perfumery practice.

Comparing Materials and Blends

Comparative evaluation is fundamental to professional judgment. Assessing materials or blends side by side reveals distinctions that guide formulation decisions. This may involve comparing the same botanical from different sources, examining a material at varying dilutions, or evaluating a blend before and after adjustment. The evaluative processes used throughout this book rely on this disciplined comparative approach.

Documentation and Olfactory Memory

Written documentation strengthens olfactory memory and supports consistency. Notes should focus on aroma, evolution, balance, longevity, and structural role. Over time, your notes become a reliable reference that sharpens accuracy and builds confidence.

Applying Nose Training to Perfume Design

Nose training underpins all perfume design work. It allows imbalance to be recognized early, structure to be evaluated accurately, and adjustments to be made intentionally, not through trial and error.

All formulation and refinement processes in this book assume the smelling, comparison, and evaluation methods established here. Training the nose is not a preliminary step, but a continuous discipline central to professional perfumery throughout a perfumer's career.

Chapter 7
Material Behavior

Perfume design is shaped as much by how materials behave as by how they smell. Every aromatic material carries a characteristic pattern of volatility, diffusion, weight, and persistence that influences how a composition unfolds over time.

Materials do not behave evenly across a perfume's lifespan. Some assert themselves immediately and fade quickly; others emerge gradually or anchor the composition for hours. Effective design accounts for these differences through deliberate distribution.

Complex materials often reveal multiple facets as they develop. Lighter components evaporate first, exposing heavier or deeper aspects later in the wear. This natural evolution can add richness and dimension, but it also introduces unpredictability. Design decisions must therefore anticipate how materials will shift, overlap, or leave gaps as the fragrance progresses.

Designing with material behavior in mind requires evaluation over time. A fragrance that feels complete at first application may thin, fragment, or lose definition as more volatile components evaporate. True performance is measured in how the composition develops after the opening—particularly in how it carries through the heart and settles into the drydown.

When materials vary in strength, persistence, or diffusion, proportional adjustment becomes necessary. This may involve reinforcing transitions, strengthening underdeveloped phases, or redistributing emphasis so that the composition maintains definition throughout its lifespan. These refinements are deliberate design decisions made to preserve clarity and continuity.

With this time–based behavior in mind, the traditional model for describing fragrance structure is the olfactory pyramid. It divides a perfume into three layers: top notes, heart notes, and base notes. Each layer plays a distinct role in how the perfume opens, develops, and lingers on the skin.

Notes, Accords, and the Olfactory Pyramid

A fragrance note refers to an individual aromatic material or impression. An accord is a combination of notes blended to create a unified aromatic idea. The olfactory pyramid organizes these notes and accords according to how quickly they evaporate.

This structure does not describe scent strength, but volatility—how fast a material rises and fades. Understanding this distinction allows the perfumer to design fragrances that are cohesive.

Top Notes: The First Impression

Top notes are the most volatile components of a perfume. They appear immediately upon application and usually fade within five to thirty minutes. Their purpose is to create the initial impression and introduce the fragrance's character.

Top notes often feel bright, fresh, or sharp. Citrus oils, light herbs, and airy aromatics commonly occupy this layer. While fleeting, top notes play an important role in shaping how a perfume is perceived at first encounter.

A successful top note does not overpower the fragrance, nor does it disappear too quickly. It prepares the wearer for what follows, guiding the transition into the heart.

Heart Notes: The Core of the Fragrance

Heart notes form the central body of the perfume. They emerge as the top notes fade and typically last several hours. This layer defines the perfume's main theme and emotional character.

Florals, spices, and aromatic herbs often dominate the heart. These materials provide continuity between the brightness of the top notes and the depth of the base. A well-designed heart note feels stable and coherent, holding the composition together.

If the heart lacks clarity, the fragrance may feel confused or unfinished.

Base Notes: Depth and Longevity

Base notes are the slowest to evaporate and linger the longest on the skin. They provide depth, warmth, and persistence, often remaining noticeable for many hours after application.

Woody materials, resins, balsams, and roots typically form the base. In addition to their scent, base notes function as fixatives, helping to anchor lighter materials and extend the life of the perfume.

When base notes are correctly balanced, they enhance the entire composition without drawing attention to themselves.

CHAPTER 8

Tools, Materials, and the Perfumer's Workspace

Understanding Perfumery Materials

Working with perfume materials requires precision, cleanliness, and an organized system for handling and documentation. While a professional laboratory is not required, a well-structured workspace protects material integrity, supports consistency, and reduces unnecessary errors during formulation.

Clean surfaces, proper ventilation, and thoughtful organization help prevent contamination and allow materials to be evaluated, stored, and used with intention.

A complete reference table classifying essential oils by note placement is provided in APPENDIX F.

Essential Blending Equipment

Specific tools form the foundation of perfume-making. Glass droppers, or pipettes, are necessary for accurately transferring essential oils. Disposable pipettes are recommended to prevent cross-contamination between oils. Graduated pipettes or syringes provide greater accuracy when working in milliliters.

Glass beakers and mixing vessels should always be used instead of plastic. Essential oils can degrade plastic and absorb unwanted odors, potentially altering the aroma of your blend. Borosilicate glass is ideal for its durability and neutrality.

A digital scale capable of measuring to at least 0.01 grams becomes increasingly important as formulas grow more complex. While counting drops may be acceptable for early experimentation, weight-based measurement ensures consistency and allows formulas to be scaled reliably.

Fragrance Blotters and Evaluation Tools

Fragrance blotters are indispensable for evaluating perfume structure. Testing on paper allows you to observe how a blend evolves without interference from skin chemistry. Blotters should be clearly labeled with the formula name and date, and stored upright while drying.

A perfumer's journal is equally important. Recording ratios, impressions, adjustments, and testing intervals transforms experimentation into intentional practice. Over time, this documentation becomes a valuable reference, helping you recognize patterns and refine your approach.

Storage and Containers

Proper storage preserves both raw materials and finished perfumes. Amber or cobalt blue glass bottles protect essential oils and blends from light exposure. Smaller bottles are ideal for test batches, while larger bottles are useful for storing finished perfumes.

All bottles should be clearly labeled with the contents, date of creation, and dilution percentage. This habit prevents confusion and ensures safety, especially when working with multiple formulations.

Perfume Bases and Carriers

Perfumes are created by diluting aromatic materials into a carrier that makes them wearable. Alcohol-based perfumes use high-proof ethanol or perfumer's alcohol, allowing the scent to diffuse quickly before settling on the skin. Oil-based perfumes use neutral carrier oils such as jojoba or fractionated coconut oil, resulting in a softer, more intimate fragrance experience.

Solid perfumes combine essential oils with beeswax and carrier oils, offering portability and longevity.

Maintaining Your Workspace

The environment in which perfume is formulated directly impacts accuracy, consistency, and sensory judgment. While safety standards are addressed in this chapter, workspace conditions determine how effectively those standards can be applied during formulation.

Adequate ventilation supports clear perception during blending by reducing olfactory fatigue and sensory overload. Proper airflow allows aromatic materials to be evaluated over longer sessions without compromising judgment, while poorly ventilated spaces increase the likelihood of distortion and over–adjustment.

Deliberate handling habits help preserve material integrity and prevent cross–contamination. Oils should be handled with intention, spills addressed promptly, and tools kept clean between uses. These practices support precision during formulation and reduce unnecessary disruption to the aromatic environment.

Blending sessions benefit from pacing. Extended exposure to concentrated aromas can dull perception and lead to overcorrection. Taking breaks and allowing the senses to reset helps ensure that formulation decisions are guided by clarity, not fatigue.

Organization within the workspace further supports accuracy. Clearly labeled bottles, clean tools, and orderly storage reduce errors and allow attention to remain on formulation, not logistics.

Raw materials should be protected from excessive heat, light, and air exposure during use. Keeping oils sealed when not in use helps maintain aromatic quality and ensures consistent performance during blending.

Alcohols Used in Perfume Making

Alcohol is a primary carrier in many perfume formats, but not all alcohols are appropriate for perfumery. When this book refers to alcohol in perfume making, it means ethanol suitable for cosmetic or fragrance use.

Appropriate alcohols for perfume formulation include perfumer's alcohol, denatured ethanol formulated specifically for fragrance use, and cosmetic-grade or food-grade ethanol, where legally permitted. These alcohols evaporate cleanly, dissolve aromatic materials effectively, and are appropriate for skin application when used correctly.

Alcohols that should not be used in perfume making include rubbing alcohol (isopropyl alcohol), surgical spirits, methanol, or any alcohol containing added fragrances, colorants, or harsh denaturants. These products can distort the fragrance, cause skin irritation, and pose safety risks.

Using the correct type of ethanol is essential for accurate scent development, safe application, and professional results.

Product Bases, Safety, and Regulatory Considerations

The base of a perfume product directly affects how a fragrance smells, performs, and wears. Alcohol, carrier oils, waxes, and bath oils each interact differently with aromatic materials, influencing diffusion, longevity, and perception. Understanding these differences is essential when formulating across multiple product formats.

Alcohol-based products emphasize volatility and projection, making top notes more prominent. Oil-based formats soften evaporation, drawing attention to heart and base notes and keeping the fragrance closer to the skin. Solid perfumes further slow diffusion, while bath and body oils require much lower concentrations to remain safe and effective. Because of these differences, the same perfume formula must be adjusted thoughtfully for each product base.

Safety considerations are inseparable from product formulation. Dilution levels must be appropriate for the intended use, application area, and frequency of exposure. Materials acceptable for fine fragrance may require lower concentrations in leave-on or whole-body products. Proper handling, accurate dilution, and clear documentation are essential professional practices.

When perfumes are created for sale, additional regulatory considerations apply. Fragrance products must comply with applicable safety standards, ingredient restrictions, and labeling requirements in the regions where they are sold. These regulations are designed to protect both consumers and makers, and they should be understood before products are offered for commercial sale.

Chapter 9
Perfume Types, Formats, and Concentrations

Perfume is defined not only by scent, but also by how it is formulated and applied. Understanding perfume types and their concentration levels helps you design fragrances suited to different preferences, occasions, and usage patterns.

Perfume Concentration Categories

Perfumes are commonly classified by the concentration of aromatic materials within the final formulation. Higher concentrations yield stronger, longer-lasting fragrances, while lower concentrations offer a more subtle experience.

Parfum, also known as extrait de parfum, contains the highest concentration of aromatic materials, typically ranging from twenty to thirty percent. These perfumes are rich, long-lasting, and require only a small amount for application.

Eau de Parfum contains slightly lower concentrations, generally around 15–20%. This format balances intensity with wearability and is one of the most popular choices for fine fragrance.

Eau de Toilette is lighter, with concentrations typically between 6% and 10%. These perfumes feel fresher and more casual, making them suitable for daily wear.

Eau de Cologne is a light fragrance format, typically containing 3–5% aromatic material. It provides a fresh, invigorating scent experience with moderate projection and relatively short wear compared to higher concentrations.

Eau Fraîche and fragrance mists are the lightest perfume formats, typically containing **1–3% aromatic materials**, and are designed to provide a soft, refreshing scent with minimal longevity.

Type	Concentration of Aromatic Compounds	Longevity
Parfum/Extrait	20–30%	8–12 hours
Eau de Parfum (EDP)	15–20%	6–8 hours
Eau de Toilette (EDT)	6–10%	4–6 hours
Eau de Cologne (EDC)	3–5%	2–4 hours
Eau Fraîche/Mist	1–3%	1–2 hours

Alcohol–Based and Oil–Based Perfumes

Alcohol–based perfumes provide immediate diffusion and clarity. The alcohol evaporates quickly, allowing the fragrance to project before settling close to the skin. This format highlights top notes and creates a traditional spray experience.

Oil–based perfumes offer a softer, more intimate effect. The carrier oil slows evaporation, allowing the fragrance to unfold gradually. Oil–based perfumes often feel warmer and more personal, with less projection but more prolonged skin contact.

Both formats have their advantages. Selection depends on design goals, not technical superiority.

Alternative Perfume Formats

Solid perfumes are created by blending aromatic materials with beeswax and carrier oils. They are portable, discreet, and long–lasting, making them well-suited for travel or subtle application.

Roll–on perfumes offer convenience and precision, allowing fragrance to be applied directly to pulse points. Hydrosol–based mists and light sprays provide a gentle aromatic experience and are often used for refreshing or seasonal blends.

Each format shapes how a fragrance is experienced. Understanding these differences allows perfumes to be designed intentionally, as opposed to adapting a formula to an unsuitable base.

How Format Changes the Way a Perfume Is Experienced

A perfume formula does not exist independently of its format. The base into which aromatic materials are diluted fundamentally shapes how a fragrance is perceived, how it moves on the skin, and how it unfolds over time.

Different product bases alter diffusion, skin presence, and perceived intensity. The rapid evaporation of ethanol allows aromatic materials—especially top notes—to lift quickly, creating clarity, projection, and immediacy. This format highlights the opening of a fragrance and allows its structure to be perceived in defined stages. Transitions between top, heart, and base notes are more apparent, making alcohol-based perfumes particularly well-suited to complex, time-based designs.

Oil-based perfumes behave differently. Carrier oils slow evaporation and compress the fragrance's structure, softening the opening and drawing attention to the heart and base. Projection is reduced, but intimacy is increased. The perfume sits closer to the skin and unfolds more gradually, often feeling warmer and more personal. Because evaporation is slower, oil-based perfumes can feel heavier at the same concentration as alcohol-based perfumes, requiring careful adjustment.

Solid perfumes further slow diffusion. The presence of wax creates a muted, grounded scent experience that prioritizes longevity and subtlety over projection. Solid formats are not intended to broadcast fragrance, but to offer a private, tactile relationship with scent. Mists and very light formats, by contrast, emphasize refreshment and atmosphere rather than structure or persistence.

A perfume is not only what it smells like—it is how it moves on the skin, how it settles over time, and how others encounter it.

Choosing a Perfume Format with Intention

Selecting a perfume format is a design decision, not a matter of convenience or personal habit. Each format supports a different kind of experience, and choosing the wrong one can distort the fragrance's intention, regardless of how well the formula is constructed.

A perfume designed for expressive projection and clarity benefits from an alcohol-based format. Fragrances built around dynamic openings, crisp transitions, or evolving structures are best experienced when volatility is allowed to occur naturally. Alcohol supports this movement and reveals the fragrance's architecture over time.

Oil-based formats are better suited to perfumes designed for closeness, warmth, and continuity. These fragrances often emphasize heart and base materials and are meant to be discovered instead of announced. In this context, reduced projection is not a flaw, but a feature that supports intimacy.

Environmental and contextual factors also influence format choice. Climate, skin type, application habits, and frequency of wear all affect how a perfume performs. A fragrance that feels balanced in an alcohol spray may feel dense in an oil roll–on, while a light composition may disappear entirely if placed in an overly subtle format.

When format is chosen intentionally, the fragrance is supported instead of constrained, and the final product feels cohesive.

Common Errors in Format and Concentration Selection

One of the most common mistakes in perfume making is assuming that higher concentration automatically produces a better or longer–lasting fragrance. In practice, excessive concentration often leads to imbalance, sensory fatigue, and diminished clarity. A perfume that is too dense may lose its ability to evolve, collapsing into a single dominant impression.

Another frequent error is applying the same concentration logic across formats. Oil–based perfumes, solids, and roll–ons maintain prolonged skin contact and therefore require more conservative aromatic percentages than alcohol–based sprays. Using extrait–level concentration in an oil format often results in heaviness, not refinement.

Beginners also commonly expect fresh or citrus–forward fragrances to perform like deep resinous perfumes. Light compositions are not designed for extended longevity; their beauty lies in immediacy and brightness. Attempting to force longevity through overconcentration or heavy fixatives often undermines the fragrance's character.

Understanding these distinctions prevents unnecessary reformulation and frustration. When concentration and format align with the fragrance's intent, the perfume performs as designed, not against its own structure.

Format as an Extension of Fragrance Identity

Format reinforces a perfume's intended presence. Some fragrances are designed to project; others are meant to remain close. When concentration and format align with purpose, the fragrance performs with clarity.

From Format to Practice

With this foundation in place, attention can now turn to the discipline that determines whether a perfume succeeds or fails: blending. The next chapter moves from conceptual decisions into practical application, examining how aromatic materials interact, support, or compete within a composition. This is where structure becomes substance, and where intentional design is transformed into a finished fragrance.

CHAPTER 10

Safety, Dilution, and Professional Standards

Working with essential oils requires knowledge, respect, and responsibility. Although these materials are natural, they are also highly concentrated aromatic substances that can cause irritation or adverse reactions if misused. When safety principles are understood and applied correctly, they allow creativity to flourish within clear and professional boundaries.

This section establishes the foundational safety practices that support responsible perfume formulation. These principles apply whether you are creating perfume for personal use, educational settings, or professional distribution.

Understanding Concentration and Dilution

Essential oils should not be applied undiluted to the skin. Appropriate dilution is a primary safety requirement in professional perfumery. Aromatic materials must be incorporated into a carrier at dermally appropriate percentages to minimize irritation, sensitization, and adverse reactions.

In practice, dilution is expressed as the percentage of aromatic materials within a finished product. These percentages must remain within safe usage thresholds based on the intended format, exposure time, and specific materials used.

From a safety perspective, concentration must be appropriate for both format and dermal exposure time. Alcohol-based sprays evaporate quickly and may tolerate higher aromatic percentages within established category norms, while oil-based and solid formats require more conservative dilution due to prolonged skin contact. Certain essential oils demand lower usage rates regardless of format because of sensitization, irritation, or phototoxic potential.

Skin Sensitivity and Patch Testing

Every individual responds differently to aromatic materials. Skin type, health status, age, and existing sensitivities influence how perfume is tolerated.

A patch test involves applying a small amount of the diluted perfume to the inside of the forearm and observing the area for twenty–four hours. If redness, itching, burning, or irritation occurs, the formulation should be adjusted or discontinued.

Some essential oils carry higher sensitization risk, particularly when used repeatedly or at elevated concentrations. Cinnamon bark, clove bud, oregano, thyme, and phenol– or aldehyde–rich oils require conservative use in perfume formulations.

In professional practice, patch testing is a standard safety protocol.

Phototoxic and Restricted Essential Oils

Certain citrus oils, particularly those expressed from the peel, contain compounds that increase the skin's sensitivity to ultra-violet light. When applied to skin and exposed to sunlight, these oils can cause phototoxic reactions such as redness, blistering, or pigmentation changes.

Phototoxic oils include, but are not limited to:

- Bergamot (expressed/cold-pressed)
- Lime (expressed/cold-pressed)
- Lemon (expressed/cold-pressed)
- Bitter orange (expressed/cold-pressed)

Steam–distilled versions of these oils are generally non–phototoxic, but confirmation from the supplier is essential. When formulating perfumes intended for daytime wear or sun exposure, phototoxic oils should be used at very low levels or avoided entirely.

Professional perfumers also remain aware of internationally recognized safety guidelines, such as those published by IFRA. IFRA guidelines provide useful maximum dermal usage references and should be consulted when formulating for sale.

Respiratory and Aromatic Exposure Awareness

Perfume making involves repeated exposure to concentrated aromas. Without proper ventilation and pacing, olfactory fatigue or respiratory irritation can occur.

Blending sessions should be kept brief, especially when working with strong base notes or resins. Taking breaks, stepping outside for fresh air, and using scent–neutralizers such as coffee beans sparingly can help reset the nose.

Respecting your own sensory limits is part of professional practice.

Labeling, Documentation, and Transparency

Clear labeling is a safety practice, not an administrative detail. Every perfume bottle should include:

- The name of the formulation
- The date of creation
- The dilution percentage
- Key aromatic materials, if shared with others

Maintaining accurate formulation records enables you to track ingredient usage, identify potential issues, and safely reproduce successful blends. In professional or educational settings, transparency builds trust and credibility.

When perfumes are shared, gifted, or sold, providing basic usage guidance and allergy disclaimers is part of ethical responsibility.

Storage and Shelf Life

Essential oils and finished perfumes should be stored in cool, dark environments away from heat and direct sunlight. Oxidation can alter aroma and increase the risk of skin irritation, particularly in citrus oils.

Finished perfumes should be monitored over time. Changes in scent, cloudiness, or irritation potential indicate degradation and signal that the product should no longer be used.

Safe storage protects both materials and users.

Safety as the Foundation of Professional Practice

Professional perfume practice requires adherence to established safety standards. Proper dilution, documentation, material awareness, and storage procedures protect both the maker and the wearer. These principles form the framework upon which all responsible perfume formulation rests.

Chapter 11
The Art of Blending

Blending is the heart of perfume making. It is where raw materials become composition, and where technical understanding meets sensory judgment.

Many beginners assume that blending is about combining pleasant-smelling oils until something agreeable emerges. In reality, effective blending is a process of managing interactions among aromatic families, chemical constituents, and evaporation rates over time. A successful blend is not defined by how many materials it contains, but by how well those materials support one another.

Blending With Purpose

One of the most common errors in perfume making is accumulation—the tendency to keep adding oils in an attempt to "fix" a blend. This often leads to muddiness, confusion, or aromatic fatigue. Each additional material introduces new constituents, new volatility patterns, and new potential conflicts.

Intentional blending begins before the first drop is added. The perfumer must decide what role the blend is meant to play. Is the fragrance intended to feel fresh and uplifting, warm and grounding, soft and floral, or deep and contemplative? Once the direction is clear, every material is evaluated not only for how it smells, but for how it behaves and what it contributes.

Effective blends often contain fewer materials than expected. When each oil has a defined purpose—lifting, rounding, anchoring, or connecting—the composition becomes clearer and more stable. Restraint is not limitation; it is precision.

Blending by Note and Structural Role

Traditional blending often organizes materials into top, heart, and base notes. While this framework provides orientation, effective blending depends on how materials function within and across these layers.

In the top phase, excessive competition creates instability. When too many volatile materials compete for attention, the opening can feel sharp or disjointed. Limiting the number of dominant top notes and assigning clear supporting roles produces a more controlled and intentional introduction.

The heart must sustain the composition once the opening dissipates. When multiple materials share similar chemical profiles—such as several ester-rich florals—the result may lack dimension. Introducing measured contrast, such as a subtle green, herbal, or lightly woody element, can restore definition and prevent monotony.

Base materials influence not only longevity but overall perception. Because heavier constituents accumulate and persist, they can easily suppress more volatile elements if overused. Excessive resins, balsams, or sesquiterpene-rich oils may reduce clarity rather than increase depth. Strategic restraint in the base often improves both diffusion and perceived balance by allowing the composition to remain open rather than congested.

Overlapping Aromatic Families and Redundancy

Redundancy occurs when multiple materials from the same aromatic family are layered without differentiation. Although the result may be harmonious, it often lacks movement, contrast, or dimensional progression.

For example, combining several florals with closely related chemical profiles can compress the heart, producing a uniform but indistinct effect. Similarly, stacking dense woods or resins may increase weight without improving depth, resulting in heaviness rather than complexity. Overlap is not inherently problematic, but it must serve a defined structural purpose.

An effective strategy is to establish a dominant family and then introduce measured contrast. A floral core may benefit from a subtle citrus lift or restrained woody support. A wood-forward composition may require a brighter opening to prevent stagnation. Controlled contrast restores articulation and prevents the composition from becoming tonally static.

Constituent Dominance and Competition

Essential oils are composed of multiple chemical constituents, and these constituents influence how oils behave together. Some constituents naturally dominate blends, even in small amounts. Phenols, aldehydes, strong ketones, and certain sesquiterpenes can easily overpower other materials.

When dominant constituents are layered without awareness, competition occurs. Rather than harmonizing, materials fight for perception. This can result in harshness, distortion, or a sense that the fragrance lacks cohesion.

For example, phenol–rich oils can overwhelm ester–rich florals, stripping them of softness. Heavy sesquiterpene–rich oils can suppress volatile top notes, preventing proper development. Cineole–heavy oils can flatten floral compositions, making them feel medicinal, not expressive.

Effective blending requires recognizing these dynamics and adjusting accordingly. Sometimes the solution is not to add another oil, but to reduce or remove one that is dominating the composition.

When Oils Cancel or Diminish One Another

Not all blending problems involve overpowering. In some cases, materials diminish one another's impact. This can happen when oils with opposing aromatic directions are combined without a bridging element, or when one oil neutralizes the perception of another.

For example, certain fresh or camphoraceous oils can mute delicate florals, while overly sweet materials can dull crisp green notes. The result is often a perfume that smells weaker or less defined than expected, despite containing potent ingredients.

Bridging materials—such as soft woods, light resins, or gentle aromatics—can restore continuity. These materials do not draw attention to themselves but connect disparate elements so the fragrance reads as a whole, not a collection of parts.

Correcting Imbalance Without Starting Over

An essential blending skill is the ability to correct a perfume without dismantling it. Many blends can be improved through measured, targeted adjustments rather than complete reformulation.

The first step is diagnosis. Does the blend feel too heavy, too sharp, too flat, or too short-lived? Identifying the dominant issue allows for precise correction. Reducing a single material by a small percentage may restore clarity more effectively than introducing additional components.

When adjustment is required, changes should be minimal and deliberate, made one at a time and evaluated over several hours. Allowing the blend to rest before intervening is equally important. Fresh compositions may integrate and soften with time, and premature modification often leads to overcorrection.

Blending as a Developing Skill

Blending skill develops through repeated practice, structured evaluation, and systematic documentation. Reviewing earlier formulations and analyzing unsuccessful trials strengthens diagnostic ability and improves future outcomes.

With experience, patterns become recognizable—materials that consistently dominate, combinations that integrate smoothly, and proportions that maintain stability. Over time, decision-making becomes more efficient and less dependent on rigid frameworks, supported instead by informed sensory judgment.

Blending proficiency is built through awareness and disciplined adjustment. Mastery arises from understanding how materials interact and applying that knowledge with consistency.

CHAPTER 12
Perfume Accords as Building Blocks

A n accord is a deliberate combination of aromatic materials designed to function as a unified scent impression. While notes refer to individual materials, accords operate as functional units within a composition.

In professional perfumery, fragrances are rarely constructed material by material from the ground up. Instead, they are developed through accords that define the fragrance's central character. This method provides greater clarity and control during formulation. For the natural perfumer, accords make it possible to create complexity from botanical materials while maintaining structural coherence.

By consolidating multiple materials into functional groups, accords reduce formulation complexity without diminishing depth. Rather than managing numerous individual oils simultaneously, the perfumer works with defined units that serve specific roles within the composition.

Understanding Accord Function

Every accord serves a defined purpose within a perfume. Some establish the primary theme, while others support structure, transition, or longevity. An accord may function as a floral heart, a woody foundation, a fresh opening, or a warm base. Regardless of its role, an effective accord should feel complete and coherent before being integrated into a larger composition.

Accords should be evaluated independently on a blotter and observed over time. If an accord collapses, becomes muddy, or shifts unpredictably on its own, those weaknesses will be amplified within the full formula. A stable accord develops in a controlled and predictable manner, maintaining clarity and structural integrity throughout its lifespan.

Horizontal Accords: Blending Within a Layer

Horizontal accords combine materials that occupy a similar evaporation range, creating breadth and density within a single structural layer.

A floral accord, for example, may blend rose, jasmine, and geranium to produce a fuller effect than any single material alone. A woody accord might combine sandalwood, cedarwood, and amyris to build texture and depth within the base.

Restraint is essential. When too many similar materials are layered, redundancy reduces clarity. The objective is not accumulation, but articulation—each material should contribute a distinct nuance such as freshness, dryness, sweetness, or warmth without duplicating another's function.

Horizontal accords benefit from measured contrast within similarity. A floral blend gains dimension when a green or lightly spicy element offsets softer notes. A woody accord becomes more dynamic when a dry wood is balanced with a creamier or subtly resinous counterpart.

Vertical Accords: Building Across Time

Vertical accords extend across top, heart, and base phases, shaping how a perfume develops over time. Rather than occupying a single layer, they guide the fragrance's progression from opening through drydown.

A citrus–floral–wood accord, for example, may open with brightness, transition into a defined floral center, and settle into a restrained woody base. Although composed of materials with differing evaporation rates, the accord reads as a continuous thematic thread.

Vertical accords are effective for smoothing transitions and maintaining thematic continuity. They reduce abrupt shifts between phases and support a coherent developmental arc.

The primary challenge lies in proportion. Materials must be weighted so that the thematic thread remains perceptible throughout development. An overemphasized base can compress progression, while an overly volatile top may fail to establish the theme. Careful testing and incremental adjustment are required.

Common Accord Categories

Certain accord types appear repeatedly in natural perfumery because they provide reliable structure and familiarity.

Floral accords often form the heart of a perfume. They may be built around a dominant flower, supported by secondary florals and modifiers that shape tone and texture. A white floral accord may feel creamy and lush, while a green floral accord feels fresh and airy.

Woody accords typically anchor a fragrance. These accords provide depth and longevity, often incorporating both dry and creamy woods. The balance between them determines whether the base feels heavy or refined.

Amber and resin accords introduce warmth and richness. Built from resins, balsams, and soft, sweet materials, these accords are powerful fixatives. They must be used with care, as even small adjustments can dramatically affect weight and projection.

Fresh accords rely on brightness and lift. Citrus, aromatic, and green materials combine to create energy and clarity. Because these materials are volatile, fresh accords often require subtle anchoring to prevent rapid fade.

Gourmand accords suggest sweetness and comfort without becoming literal. In natural perfumery, these effects are achieved through resins, absolutes, and warm spices.

Accords as Modular Design Elements

A primary advantage of working with accords is modularity. Once an accord has been stabilized and characterized, it can be adapted across multiple formulations. This approach supports stylistic continuity while allowing controlled variation.

An established accord may be adjusted to suit different applications. A floral accord, for example, can be lightened through brighter supporting materials or deepened through restrained base reinforcement, depending on the intended format or context.

Modular design is standard practice in professional perfumery. Over time, a perfumer may develop a set of core accords that function as recurring structural elements within their work.

Evaluating and Refining Accords

Accords should be evaluated as rigorously as finished perfumes. They should be tested on blotter and skin, observed over several hours, and documented carefully. An accord that smells complete at first may reveal weaknesses in the later stages of wear that require adjustment.

Refinement is often achieved through reduction. Removing a material that introduces noise or redundancy can clarify the accord more effectively than expanding the formula. Small ratio changes frequently produce significant improvements.

Accords should be allowed to rest before final evaluation. Aging supports integration and reveals whether the accord is structurally stable. Rushing this process often introduces instability into the final perfume.

Accords as the Framework of Perfume

Accords shift blending from sequential material addition to structured composition. They move the focus from individual components to functional units that shape development and coherence. Mastery of accord construction allows complexity to be managed with precision and control.

A consolidated visual reference of horizontal and vertical accord structure is provided in APPENDIX I.

CHAPTER 13
Defining Intention Before Formulating

Before advancing into full construction and finalized formulas, it is necessary to define how the perfume is expected to perform in use. Effective fragrance design begins prior to material selection, with decisions about projection, longevity, context, and intended experience.

This step does not involve assigning functional claims or predicting outcomes. It establishes the practical parameters that will inform subsequent formulation decisions. When these parameters are defined clearly, material selection becomes more efficient and revision more deliberate.

Clarifying the Role of the Fragrance

Begin by defining how the fragrance should exist within the wearer's environment:

- Should it project immediately or emerge gradually?

- Should it remain subtle and supportive, or assert a defined presence?
- Is it designed for habitual daily wear or for occasional, deliberate use?

These distinctions directly influence diffusion, contrast, and density. A composition intended for frequent wear typically requires restraint and controlled projection, whereas a fragrance designed for specific moments may accommodate greater intensity or structural complexity.

Considering Time and Presence

Next, define how the fragrance should develop over time:

- Should the opening be brief and restrained, or extended and pronounced?
- Is continuity prioritized over contrast?
- Should the drydown remain intimate, or maintain perceptible projection?

These decisions determine the proportion of volatile and persistent materials, the construction of accords, and the pacing of development. Consistency in formulation depends on understanding both duration and progression.

Context Shapes Structure

Fragrance is experienced within a specific context. Environment influences whether a composition feels appropriate or intrusive.

Consider:

- Where will the fragrance most often be worn?
- What competing sensory inputs are present in that setting?
- What proximity will the wearer have to others?

Close-contact environments typically require restrained diffusion and moderated contrast. Open or spacious settings may accommodate greater lift and clarity to maintain perceptibility without excess density.

Translating Intention Into Structure

Once the design parameters are established, formulation choices follow logically:

- Proportion establishes weight and emphasis
- Accord construction governs coherence and transition
- Diffusion controls projection and skin presence
- Drydown influences longevity and residual impression

Material selection should follow these structural requirements. Rather than beginning with traditionally associated ingredients, define the desired performance first and select materials accordingly.

Designing With Restraint

Functional fragrance design requires restraint. Conceptual alignment alone does not justify inclusion, and not every effect warrants emphasis. Clarity is frequently achieved through reduction rather than expansion.

When the objective is defined precisely, completion becomes easier to identify. Excess becomes apparent, and adjustments can be made with intention and control.

With the design parameters defined, formulation can proceed into structured construction. The next chapter translates these decisions into the development of an aromatic concentrate.

CHAPTER 14

Formulation Method: From Concept to Concentrate

With the design parameters defined, the work shifts from planning to building. This chapter presents a clear method for turning those decisions into a structured aromatic concentrate. The focus is on proportion, sequencing, and precise dilution so that each formula can be evaluated, adjusted, and reproduced with consistency.

Designing the Perfume as a 100–Drop (or 100–Part) Concentrate

In professional perfumery, a fragrance is first developed as a complete aromatic concentrate—often referred to in industry as the "juice." This concentrate represents 100% of the aromatic composition prior to dilution.

Working in this format allows the perfumer to refine proportion and accord relationships independently of product base. Top, heart, and base materials are calculated so that the formula totals 100 parts, creating a controlled and measurable framework. Once finalized, the concentrate can be diluted into different perfume formats without altering its core identity.

Accords as the Foundation of Perfume Design

In practice, perfumes are developed from accords rather than isolated materials. Each phase—top, heart, and base—is first built as a functional unit before being integrated into the complete composition.

Working in this way supports clarity and control during formulation, allowing each component to be evaluated independently before contributing to the finished fragrance.

Structural Proportions and Variations

Classic perfume architecture often follows approximate proportions of 20–30% top, 40–50% heart, and 20–30% base. These ratios provide a practical starting point for many compositions.

In professional practice, however, formulas are adapted to suit design objectives. Some incorporate bridge materials to smooth transitions, while others use modifiers in small percentages to refine texture or tonal direction. Resinous or extract-style perfumes may minimize traditional top notes, whereas very fresh compositions may emphasize the opening with reduced base support.

These guidelines serve as a foundation, not a fixed formula.

Dilution into Different Perfume Types

The aromatic concentrate functions as the structural blueprint for the fragrance and forms the basis for evaluation and refinement. Once finalized, it is diluted according to the intended product format. Standard concentration ranges are outlined below. Detailed dilution calculations and volume conversion charts are provided in APPENDIX A.

Extrait de Parfum (20–30%):

Use 20–30% of the aromatic concentrate.

Eau de Parfum (15–20%):

Use 15–20% of the aromatic concentrate.

Eau de Toilette (6–10%):

Use 6–10% of the aromatic concentrate.

Eau de Cologne (3–5%):

Use 3–5% of the aromatic concentrate.

Eau Faîche (1–3%):

Use 1–3% of the aromatic concentrate.

The percentages above represent the proportion of aromatic concentrate within the final diluted product. The remainder of the product consists of perfumer's alcohol (or other appropriate base) brought to the desired final volume.

Professional Dilution of Perfume Materials (Using Scales)

Professional perfume formulation relies on weight-based measurement to ensure accuracy, repeatability, and consistency across batches. Drop size varies according to viscosity, dropper design, and ambient conditions, making drop counting unreliable for precise work. Measuring by weight removes these variables and allows formulas to be reproduced reliably.

Dilution serves both safety and formulation control. Pre-diluting materials provides finer adjustment of proportion, particularly when working with potent essential oils, absolutes, or materials used at trace levels. Selecting an appropriate dilution strength improves control and reduces the risk of over-concentration.

A 10% dilution is suitable for many materials during formula construction. Highly concentrated or intense materials are often more manageable at 1%, allowing accurate measurement without overwhelming the blend.

Use a digital scale accurate to at least 0.01 g. To prepare 10 g of a 10% dilution, combine 1 g of aromatic material with 9 g of diluent. To prepare 10 g of a 1% dilution, combine 0.1 g of material with 9.9 g of diluent.

Viscous materials and certain absolutes may require gentle warming in a water bath to incorporate fully. Heat only briefly and avoid excessive temperature to preserve aromatic quality.

Step–by–Step Method for Making a Perfume

The steps below describe the sequence for constructing an aromatic concentrate. They do not cover the full evaluation, aging, or final product workflow.

1. **Define the intended product format and container.** The aromatic concentrate will be built independently of dilution, but the intended format informs design constraints (projection, exposure time, and concentration limits).
2. **Define the fragrance direction.** Specify the overall character and presence (e.g., fresh, soft, warm, deep) and how it should be experienced in use.
3. **Select the fragrance family or families.** Establish a dominant family and a supporting secondary family if needed.
4. **Set target proportions.** Use the classic top/heart/base framework as a starting point and adjust to suit the intended style and performance.
5. **Build the top, heart, and base accords.** Evaluate each accord independently before integration.
6. **Blend in sequence.** Combine heart first, then base, then top, refining proportions as needed.
7. **Select dilution for the finished product.** Once the concentrate is finalized, dilute according to the intended product type.

A complete start–to–finish workflow—including rest time, evaluation, and product execution—is presented in Chapter 18.

Demonstration: One Perfume Formula Expressed Across Perfume Types

The Perfume Formula — 100 Drops Total

This example illustrates how a perfume is constructed as a complete aromatic concentrate before dilution or product format is applied. The 100–drop model makes proportional relationships visible and allows the same formula to be translated across multiple perfume types without altering its internal ratios. Once established, the concentrate can be diluted into extrait, eau de parfum, or other formats while preserving the intended design.

Although professional production relies on weight-based measurement, the 100–drop model is used here solely to demonstrate proportional structure clearly.

Top Accord – 25% (25 drops)

Bergamot 15 drops (15%)

Sweet Orange 10 drops (10%)

Heart Accord – 45% (45 drops)

Lavender 20 drops (20%)

Geranium 15 drops (15%)

Clary Sage 10 drops (10%)

Base Accord – 30% (30 drops)

Cedarwood 15 drops (15%)

Frankincense 10 drops (10%)

Vetiver 5 drops (5%)

The total equals 100 drops, ensuring proportional clarity before dilution.

Chapter 15
Advanced Accord Structures

Once basic accord construction is understood, the next level involves controlling how accords function within the complete composition. Advanced structures address not only how materials combine, but how they project, anchor, and develop across the lifespan of the perfume. At this stage, formulation shifts from simple assembly to coordinated design.

At this level, performance characteristics distinguish a casual blend from a composed fragrance. Expansion, compression, persistence, and projection are shaped through proportion and accord placement. These outcomes result from deliberate design decisions made during construction.

Vertical Architecture and Time–Based Design

Vertical architecture describes how related accords are distributed across the lifespan of a perfume. The fragrance is designed as a continuous progression, with each phase guiding perception from the opening through the drydown.

A vertically integrated composition often features related materials across multiple layers. A citrus–wood theme, for example, may open with bright citrus notes, move into a citrus–inflected floral heart, and settle into a softly resinous woody base. Although the materials shift, the aromatic theme remains recognizable. This continuity prevents abrupt transitions as the perfume develops.

Vertical design demands careful proportion. If the base expression is weighted too heavily, it can compress the progression and mute earlier phases. If the top expression is overly volatile, the theme may fade before it is fully established. Effective vertical construction maintains thematic presence while allowing natural development.

Diffusion, Projection, and Sillage

Diffusion describes how a fragrance radiates from the skin, while sillage refers to the trail it leaves behind. These characteristics are shaped primarily at the accord level rather than by isolated materials.

Certain materials project more readily, particularly lighter, volatile components found in citrus oils, aromatic herbs, and some florals. Others remain closer to the skin, contributing warmth and depth without strong projection. Advanced blending involves pairing these materials deliberately so diffusion feels controlled rather than accidental.

An accord designed for stronger projection must remain composed. Excessive diffusion can produce sharpness or sensory fatigue, while overly dense accords may feel compressed or muted. Adjusting diffusion often requires reducing excess weight rather than increasing brightness. Creating space within the composition can enhance both projection and persistence.

Fixative Accords and Longevity Control

Longevity in natural perfumery is frequently misunderstood. It is not achieved by simply increasing heavy base materials, but by constructing fixative accords that stabilize the composition as a whole. While many fixatives originate in the base, not all base materials function as true fixatives; they are selected specifically for their ability to slow evaporation and reinforce persistence.

Fixative accords commonly combine woods, resins, and balsamic materials in proportions that anchor volatile elements without masking them. By moderating evaporation, these accords extend wear time while maintaining continuity.

An effective fixative accord remains understated. Its influence should be perceived through stability rather than distinct prominence. When overemphasized, fixatives reduce transparency and create density. When proportioned carefully, they increase longevity while preserving clarity.

Structural Transitions and Bridging Materials

Transitions between accords are critical moments in a perfume's development. Abrupt shifts can feel disjointed, while gradual transitions create continuity and ease. Bridging materials support these transitions by sharing characteristics across adjacent accords.

For example, a floral heart may move more seamlessly into a woody base when a lightly woody or resin-tinged floral is incorporated. These materials do not dominate the composition; they moderate contrast and guide progression.

Because bridging materials rarely stand out, they are often undervalued. Yet they play a central role in maintaining cohesion. Without them, a fragrance may feel segmented rather than integrated.

Weight, Transparency, and Density

Advanced accord design requires managing perceived weight. Weight describes how heavy or light a fragrance feels, independent of intensity. A perfume may project strongly yet remain airy, or feel subdued yet dense.

Density increases when heavier materials overlap, particularly within the base. Lightness emerges when space is preserved between components, even at higher concentrations. Skilled perfumers adjust perceived weight through proportion and selective reduction rather than relying solely on dilution.

In natural perfumery, this control is especially important. Botanical materials are inherently complex, and preserving space within the composition allows nuance to remain perceptible rather than congested.

Refining Structure Through Reduction

At advanced stages, refinement frequently involves removal rather than addition. Reducing an accord to its essential components often clarifies form and improves overall performance. This approach requires restraint and decisive evaluation.

A practical technique is to temporarily remove one material from an accord and observe the change. In many cases, the composition gains clarity, indicating that the omitted material was contributing redundancy rather than support.

Reduction reinforces precision. Each remaining material should serve a defined function within the composition.

Structural Consistency Across a Collection

For perfumers developing multiple fragrances, advanced accord structures support continuity across a body of work. Reusing foundational accords in varied proportions or contexts creates a recognizable style without duplication.

This method allows exploration within a defined framework. Each perfume remains distinct yet related. Over time, this cohesion becomes part of the perfumer's signature.

Advanced Structure as the Foundation of Mastery

Mastery in perfumery is demonstrated through control rather than complexity. Advanced accord structures provide control over progression, proportion, and projection, allowing fragrances to remain composed and intentional throughout their development.

With these principles established, the focus now shifts to applying them in the construction of an original perfume—from initial concept through finished blend.

For a consolidated reference of material roles and performance behavior, see APPENDIX H.

CHAPTER 16
Designing a Perfume with Purpose

Designing an original perfume is a structured process that transforms an idea into a wearable composition. While intuition informs creative direction, successful design depends on clear parameters, measured construction, and systematic refinement. This chapter moves from theory into application, outlining the steps required to translate concept into finished fragrance.

Effective design begins with defined objectives. Without a clear direction, blends tend to accumulate materials without coherence. When the intended character and use of the fragrance are established from the outset, formulation becomes more focused and adjustments become more precise.

Defining the Concept and Emotional Direction

Every perfume begins with a defined idea. This may originate from a mood, season, environment, or sensory impression. The concept does not need to be elaborate, but it must be specific enough to guide material selection and proportion.

Clarifying the intended direction determines fragrance family, weight, and overall construction. A composition intended to feel fresh and energizing requires different materials and balance than one designed to feel warm or contemplative. Writing a brief concept statement provides a reference point during formulation and helps prevent unnecessary deviation.

The concept also informs format and concentration decisions. A light, daily fragrance may be better suited to an eau de toilette or oil–based roll–on, while a denser composition may benefit from a higher concentration.

Selecting Fragrance Direction

Once the concept is established, the next step is selecting a clear fragrance direction. This involves identifying the dominant fragrance family and defining the overall compositional emphasis.

At this stage, the perfumer determines whether the fragrance will be floral–forward, woody–centered, fresh, resinous, or a hybrid expression. This decision narrows the working palette and reduces unnecessary experimentation. The intended time progression is also considered—whether the composition will emphasize a pronounced heart, sustained base presence, or an expressive opening.

Establishing this framework early prevents imbalance during construction. When the intended form is defined in advance, materials are chosen for their function rather than introduced reactively.

Building the Initial Formula

The first formula is not the finished perfume; it is a working draft that establishes proportion and interaction between materials. Construction typically begins with the heart, as this layer defines the fragrance's core character.

Once the heart is balanced, base materials are introduced to provide support and persistence. Top notes are added last, shaping the opening without disturbing the central theme. Working in this sequence promotes stability during early construction.

At this stage, restraint is essential. Limiting the number of materials allows clearer observation of behavior and easier diagnosis of imbalance. Additional complexity can be introduced once the foundation performs reliably.

Working in Ratios and Proportions

Proportion determines performance more than individual materials. A perfume succeeds or fails based on balance and interaction within the formula. Understanding ratio allows adjustments to be made without destabilizing the composition.

Even minor modifications can produce significant effects. Increasing or reducing a dominant material by a small amount may alter the entire balance. For this reason, adjustments should be incremental and carefully documented.

Measuring by weight rather than drops improves precision and repeatability. As formulas advance toward final refinement, weight–based measurement ensures accurate replication and reliable scaling.

Iteration and Controlled Adjustment

Perfume design is iterative. Most formulas require multiple versions before they resolve, and each version provides information that guides the next adjustment.

After blending, evaluate the perfume on blotter and skin over several hours. Record observations at defined intervals to track development, transitions, and longevity. Issues such as heaviness, sharpness, or collapse typically appear during this stage rather than in the opening.

Adjustments should be controlled and specific. Change one element at a time so cause and effect remain clear.

Knowing When to Refine and When to Rest

One of the most challenging aspects of perfume design is recognizing when a formula is complete. Over-adjustment can introduce new imbalance and obscure the original direction.

Allowing a perfume to rest before making changes is often beneficial. Aging enables materials to integrate, softening rough edges and revealing the composition more clearly. Many formulas improve after several days—or even weeks—of rest.

If the fragrance fulfills its original objective, develops well over time, and remains balanced, additional modification may not be warranted. Restraint protects clarity.

Developing Confidence in Original Design

Original perfume design is not driven by comparison, but by alignment with defined creative objectives. Over time, patterns emerge in material selection, compositional tendencies, and preferred effects.

Recognizing these patterns contributes to stylistic consistency. Professional confidence develops through repeated practice, documentation, and informed evaluation.

Chapter 17

Evaluation, Refinement, and Iteration

Evaluation is where perfume design becomes measurable. A blend may seem promising at first application, but its true performance is revealed through timed observation and controlled adjustment. This chapter outlines how to assess a fragrance systematically, identify imbalance, and refine a formula without destabilizing it.

Refinement is not about adding complexity; it is about ensuring that the fragrance performs as intended. A formula is considered refined when it develops predictably from opening through drydown, maintains balance on the skin, and remains consistent with its original objective.

Initial Evaluation: First Impression Versus Performance

The first impression of a perfume is informative but not conclusive. Fresh blends often smell disjointed or sharp, with volatile materials dominating while base components remain subdued. Evaluating too quickly can lead to unnecessary adjustments and overcorrection.

Early assessment should focus on identifying major concerns rather than subtle nuances. Does the opening feel harsh or unfocused? Is the overall direction clear? Is any material immediately overpowering? These observations inform later refinement but should not prompt immediate reformulation.

Allow the perfume to rest for at least twenty–four hours before conducting a full evaluation. This interval permits integration and provides a more accurate representation of performance.

Blotter Testing: Observing Structure Without Skin Influence

Fragrance blotters provide a neutral surface for evaluating progression without the variability of skin chemistry. Label each strip clearly with the formula name and date.

Assess the perfume at defined intervals—such as 15 minutes, 1 hour, 3 hours, and 6 hours. Record how the fragrance transitions, whether any phase feels abrupt or compressed, and how long it remains perceptible.

Blotter testing reveals issues such as uneven transitions, imbalance between phases, or premature fade. It is particularly useful for assessing early development and overall continuity.

Skin Testing: Evaluating Wearability and Interaction

Skin testing reveals how a perfume responds to warmth, moisture, and individual chemistry. Apply a small amount to pulse points and observe its development over several hours.

Assess projection, skin presence, and whether any materials become irritating or unpleasant with wear. Some components that perform well on blotter may shift on skin—appearing sharper, sweeter, or heavier than expected.

Testing on multiple individuals highlights variability in performance and perception. While a fragrance does not need universal approval, understanding its range of behavior supports responsible refinement.

Identifying Common Structural Problems

Many formulation issues follow recognizable patterns. Learning to diagnose them allows efficient correction.

A perfume that feels flat frequently contains excessive overlap within a single aromatic family. Reducing redundancy or introducing controlled contrast typically restores dimension. A fragrance that feels heavy or oppressive often relies too heavily on base materials, limiting volatility and progression.

Short-lived perfumes usually lack adequate support. Strengthening transitions or incorporating a subtle fixative accord often improves longevity more effectively than increasing overall concentration.

Harsh openings commonly result from imbalance within the top layer or excessive volatile materials. Reducing these elements, rather than attempting to mask them, typically yields cleaner results.

Corrective Techniques and Targeted Adjustment

Refinement should be deliberate and incremental. Once an issue is identified, adjustments should address the underlying cause rather than masking symptoms.

Reduction is often the most effective correction. A small decrease in a dominant material can significantly improve clarity and balance. If addition is required, it should be minimal and introduced one change at a time.

Avoid modifying multiple variables simultaneously. Doing so obscures cause and effect and reduces the reliability of evaluation. Each adjustment should be tested, recorded, and reassessed before further changes are made.

Aging and Integration

Time plays a critical role in perfume refinement. Aging allows materials to integrate more fully, clarifying their interaction within the composition. Many formulas soften, deepen, and stabilize after several days or weeks.

Observe aged perfumes for changes in aroma, clarity, and skin response. Resting can reveal concerns not apparent in fresh blends, including oxidation or imbalance within heavier materials.

A fragrance that improves with aging is generally well-constructed. One that degrades or becomes unstable may require adjustment or reconsideration of specific components.

Knowing When a Perfume Is Finished

A perfume is complete when it fulfills its defined objective, performs consistently over time, and remains balanced without requiring continued correction. Determining this point requires disciplined evaluation supported by experience.

Perfection is neither attainable nor necessary. Excessive modification often diminishes clarity and character without improving performance. When additional changes no longer address a specific issue, the formula has reached resolution.

A fragrance cannot be refined indefinitely. Repeated, uncertain adjustments introduce instability rather than improvement. Professional practice prioritizes coherence and performance over flawlessness. A finished perfume is defined by reliable function in use.

Documentation and Learning Through Evaluation

Each evaluation generates information that extends beyond a single formula. Systematic documentation of observations, adjustments, and outcomes builds a working reference that strengthens future development.

Over time, patterns become clear—materials that consistently dominate, combinations that integrate reliably, and proportions that produce stable performance. This accumulated data reduces unnecessary experimentation and improves efficiency.

Evaluation is not separate from formulation; it informs it. Through consistent observation and controlled refinement, skill develops through measurable experience.

Chapter 18
Developing a Signature Design Language

A signature design language is not a single perfume, nor is it defined by a preferred ingredient. It is a consistent approach to proportion, material selection, diffusion, and development. While individual compositions may vary in style or family, recognizable continuity emerges from repeated structural decisions rather than repeated formulas.

A signature develops gradually once foundational skills are established. It cannot be imposed prematurely or manufactured through preference alone. Instead, it becomes evident through documented patterns in formulation, evaluation, and refinement. This chapter examines how to identify those patterns and refine them without limiting range.

Recognizing Patterns in Your Work

The first step in developing a functional signature is systematic observation. When finished perfumes are reviewed collectively, patterns begin to emerge. These patterns may appear in recurring fragrance families, frequently selected materials, or consistent compositional decisions.

Common preferences may include:

- Smooth rather than dramatic openings
- Moderate diffusion instead of strong projection
- Gradual transitions rather than abrupt shifts
- A consistent approach to weight, transparency, or pacing

These tendencies are not flaws to correct; they indicate how you naturally construct fragrance. Identify which perfumes feel most resolved and perform most reliably. Note recurring adjustments made during refinement. These repeated decisions form the basis of a recognizable design approach.

Thorough documentation is essential. Written evaluation enables objective comparison across multiple formulas and reveals consistent tendencies in practice.

Evaluating Structural Completion and Balance

One of the more challenging aspects of advanced perfumery is recognizing when a formula has reached resolution. Completion is not defined by the number of materials or the appearance of complexity, but by functional cohesion within the composition.

A resolved perfume demonstrates internal consistency. Each material serves a defined role, and no component exists merely to compensate for imbalance elsewhere. The fragrance develops predictably and maintains clarity through its progression. When further adjustments no longer produce measurable improvement, the formula has reached its endpoint.

Signs a Structure Is Complete

- The opening, heart, and drydown transition smoothly without sharp breaks
- No single material dominates unless intentionally designed to do so
- Removing any one material weakens the structure rather than clarifying it
- The composition remains stable across multiple wears and formats
- Further adjustments produce lateral change without improvement

Signs You Are Overworking a Formula

- Loss of clarity in the opening after repeated adjustments
- Increasing muddiness or flattening instead of added dimension
- Reliance on trace additions to "fix" the balance instead of addressing the proportion
- Escalating complexity without a corresponding increase in coherence

Structural Imbalance vs. Material Imbalance

Structural imbalance is indicated when:

- The perfume collapses too quickly or lingers without resolution
- Transitions feel rushed, stalled, or uneven
- Adjustments to individual materials fail to correct the issue

Material imbalance is indicated when:

- A specific material consistently overpowers the composition
- One note disrupts harmony regardless of dosage
- Removing or replacing a single material restores clarity

Common Structural Failure Modes in Natural Perfume

Even well–constructed formulas can fail when structural relationships are misunderstood or pushed beyond their limits. Recognizing common failure modes allows the perfumer to diagnose problems early and correct them through proportion and architectural adjustment rather than adding more materials.

One frequent failure is structural collapse, in which the perfume opens with promise but quickly loses coherence. This often results from insufficient anchoring, overemphasis on volatile materials, or imbalance between the opening and its underlying support. The solution is rarely to add more base notes, but to reassess proportional weight and continuity.

Another common issue is muddiness, in which individual materials lose definition and the composition reads as flat or blurred. Muddiness typically arises from excessive layering of materials with similar profiles or from attempting to correct imbalance through accumulation instead of simplification. Simplification often restores clarity more effectively than replacement.

Over–anchoring occurs when heavy materials dominate, slowing development and obscuring transitions. In these cases, the perfume may feel dense or static, with little evolution over time. Correction requires reducing weight or redistributing materials so that diffusion and pacing are restored.

A subtler failure is directional confusion, in which a perfume lacks a clear center or trajectory. This can occur when multiple accords compete for attention or when supporting materials are not clearly subordinated. Strengthening a central accord and reducing secondary distractions helps reestablish focus.

Finally, volatility imbalance can cause a perfume to feel either fleeting or overwhelming. When evaporation rates across materials are poorly aligned, the composition may rush through the opening or linger unresolved. Correction requires recalibrating proportions to restore coherent progression.

Understanding and Articulating Design Choices

As skill advances, design is defined less by what is included and more by why it is selected. The ability to articulate these decisions—internally or in writing—marks the shift from competent formulation to intentional design.

Every formula reflects exclusion as much as inclusion. Selecting one material over another may depend on volatility, weight, transparency, or functional role within an accord. A resin may be chosen for continuity rather than depth, or a floral for lift rather than prominence. These decisions influence performance as much as aroma.

During formulation, targeted questions clarify purpose:

- What functional role does this material serve?
- What changes if it is reduced, replaced, or removed?
- Does it reinforce the central direction, or compensate for imbalance?

Effective formulas demonstrate economy. Materials are selected to perform defined tasks, not because they are familiar or appealing in isolation. When a choice improves clarity, pacing, or cohesion, it earns its place. When it does not, reduction is preferable.

This awareness enables refinement without unnecessary expansion. Over time, consistent decision patterns become visible, revealing a coherent design logic that can be applied across compositions.

Structural Review During Formulation

During formulation, there are key stages at which structural review is essential. These moments prevent overworking, premature refinement, and progress built on unstable foundations. Review should occur during construction—not after failure—as a deliberate assessment of how the composition behaves before moving forward.

After Establishing the Initial Framework

At this stage, the perfume should present a readable opening and a clear direction.

A formula built around multiple bright citrus materials—such as lemon, bergamot, and grapefruit—may feel lively but unfocused if they compete at equal intensity. When the opening smells sharp yet indistinct, competition within the same volatility range is usually the cause.

Another common pattern is an opening dominated by green or aromatic materials that feels crisp at first but disappears within minutes. This often reflects insufficient continuity between the opening and what follows—not a need for heavier base notes.

If the opening feels busy, simplify.

If it fades too quickly, strengthen continuity before introducing new material.

Before Refining Transitions

Transitions should be supported by proportion, not patched through accumulation.

A floral heart composed of several soft florals—such as lavender, geranium, and rose—may smell pleasant yet unstable if none anchors the center. When smoothness requires repeated trace corrections, the imbalance lies in hierarchy and proportion.

Another issue arises when a resin or wood is added to smooth a transition but instead flattens the heart. In this case, the supporting material competes rather than reinforces.

If transitions require repeated correction, reassess proportion and hierarchy instead of layering additional materials.

Before Finalizing the Formula

A finished composition should resolve without collapse or stagnation.

A drydown that feels thin or hollow often results from insufficient continuity among lighter woods or resins. Adding heavier materials may increase persistence but rarely restores coherence.

Conversely, a drydown dominated by dense resins or heavy woods can feel static, as though development has stopped. This usually indicates over-anchoring rather than completion.

A resolved perfume maintains identity through the drydown while allowing a natural conclusion.

Before Scaling or Adapting Formats

Stability must be confirmed before expansion.

If a perfume smells clear immediately after blending but becomes muddled after resting, this often indicates unresolved proportion between materials of similar weight—commonly florals layered with soft woods or resins.

Another warning sign is inconsistency across evaluations despite stable conditions. Weak proportion frequently reveals itself through unpredictability over time.

Do not scale or adapt a formula until it performs consistently across repeated assessments.

Formulation Self–Assessment Table

Observed Behavior	Likely Structural Cause	What to Check First	Corrective Action
Opening smells sharp but unfocused	Too many materials competing at the same volatility level	Number of top materials and their relative proportions	Reduce competing materials; establish a clear hierarchy

Observed Behavior	Likely Structural Cause	What to Check First	Corrective Action
Opening smells pleasant but disappears quickly	Weak continuity between volatile and supporting materials	Relationship between top and heart proportions	Strengthen connective materials rather than adding base weight
Heart smells smooth but indistinct	No clear central accord	Whether one material or accord carries the center	Simplify and reinforce the core accord
Heart requires repeated trace fixes	Core imbalance masked by modifiers	Frequency and purpose of trace adjustments	Return to core proportions; remove corrective layers
Transitions feel abrupt or uneven	Misaligned pacing between sections	Proportional relationship between heart and base	Adjust ratios to smooth progression
Drydown feels thin or hollow	Continuity gap rather than lack of weight	Link between heart-to-base materials over time	Improve continuity before adding density
Drydown feels heavy or static	Over–anchoring	Dominance of dense materials	Reduce weight; restore lift and pacing

Observed Behavior	Likely Structural Cause	What to Check First	Corrective Action
Perfume smells clear one day, muddled the next	Unresolved overlap among similar–weight materials	Layering of florals, woods, or resins	Simplify and rebalance before further refinement
Formula changes character after resting	Instability revealed over time	Performance after rest vs. fresh impression	Pause adjustments; reassess proportions and hierarchy
Adjustments no longer improve the perfume	Formula has reached resolution	Whether changes produce improvement or only variation	Stop adjusting; document final performance

Consistency Without Repetition

A functional signature is built on consistent principles rather than repeated outcomes. You may work across different fragrance families or formats, yet your compositions remain recognizable because the underlying design approach follows a familiar logic.

Consistency often appears in:

- How top, heart, and base are proportioned
- How density and diffusion are controlled

- How transitions and drydown are shaped
- How restrained or expansive the overall composition feels

Recurring accords reinforce this continuity. A foundational woody, resinous, or aromatic accord may be adapted across perfumes while preserving design identity. Likewise, returning to established proportional relationships supports coherence without duplicating scent.

The objective is recognizability through method, not uniformity.

Refinement as a Design Skill

As a signature takes shape, refinement becomes more important than experimentation. Refinement is the discipline of deciding what does not belong. Removing materials, effects, or habitual patterns that dilute clarity strengthens the work.

For some perfumers, refinement means simplifying formulas and reducing overlap. For others, it means managing complexity while preserving transparency. Neither direction is inherently superior. What matters is consistency between intention and outcome.

At this stage, each material must justify its place. Adjustments are deliberate, not reactive.

Signature as Functional Voice

A functional fragrance signature becomes recognizable through consistent design decisions. Recognition develops not from a single note, but from how a composition unfolds, settles, and maintains presence over time.

This consistency is strengthened through confidence in evaluation and refinement methods. When adjustments are guided by clear criteria rather than uncertainty, formulas become more cohesive and deliberate.

A strong signature does not depend on universal appeal. Its value lies in clarity of direction and reliability in execution. Consistent design choices give the work a distinct and stable identity.

Maintaining Growth Within a Signature Framework

Developing a signature does not restrict growth; it provides a consistent foundation for intentional expansion. Growth emerges through deeper familiarity with materials, subtle shifts in proportion and pacing, and the careful introduction of new elements.

New materials can be incorporated within established design relationships. New formats can be explored without disrupting compositional continuity. These measured adjustments keep the work dynamic without compromising stability.

A functional signature supports exploration while maintaining coherence.

Signature as Professional Foundation

For perfumers working professionally or teaching others, a clear signature provides continuity and credibility. It allows others to recognize your approach and understand what defines your work.

Even in personal practice, a signature serves as a reference point. It reflects not only technical ability but also design maturity—the result of experience shaping decisions over time.

A fragrance signature is not a fixed endpoint. It evolves as skill deepens. What remains consistent is not a specific perfume, but the method behind its construction.

CHAPTER 19
Perfume Formats in Practice

Once a perfume has been designed, evaluated, and refined, the next consideration is how it will be worn. Delivery method significantly influences how a fragrance is perceived. Alcohol-based sprays, roll-ons, solids, and layered applications each affect diffusion, longevity, and skin presence—even when the aromatic composition remains unchanged.

Understanding delivery mechanics allows the perfumer to adapt a formula deliberately rather than treating presentation as an afterthought. A well-constructed fragrance should feel complete within its chosen format, with proportion and balance adjusted to suit how it is applied.

Eau de Parfum Formulation in Practice

Eau de parfum is one of the most versatile formats, balancing strength with wearability. It offers noticeable projection without overwhelming the wearer. In this format, the opening is more pronounced, followed by a defined heart and a supportive base.

When formulating for eau de parfum, volatility must be managed carefully. Bright top notes should be proportioned so they do not dissipate too quickly, exposing the heart prematurely. Base materials must provide support without adding unnecessary density.

Because alcohol enhances diffusion, accords that felt balanced in oil may require recalibration. Base materials can often be reduced slightly, as projection compensates for perceived weight. Final ratios should always be tested within the intended format before completion.

Oil–Based Roll–On Perfumes

Oil–based perfumes offer a more intimate scent experience. They sit closer to the skin and unfold gradually, making them ideal for personal fragrance or situations where subtlety is preferred.

Because oil slows evaporation, heart and base notes are emphasized more strongly than top notes. As a result, formulas designed for oil–based applications often require brighter or more defined openings to avoid feeling heavy or muted.

Roll–on perfumes benefit from clarity and restraint. Overly complex blends can feel dense in oil form. Reducing redundancy and focusing on smooth transitions enhances wearability.

Solid Perfume Design

Solid perfumes combine aromatic materials with beeswax and carrier oils, creating a portable and long-lasting format. The wax adds weight and warmth, influencing how the fragrance develops on the skin.

In solid perfumes, volatility is reduced further. This makes them ideal for woody, resinous, or gourmand-style fragrances, while very light or citrus-forward perfumes may lose definition.

When designing for solid format, the perfumer must account for the wax's influence. Slightly increasing brightness or contrast within the accord structure can prevent dullness. Solid perfumes should be tested over extended wear periods to assess longevity and clarity.

Layering and Modular Use

Layering involves applying multiple perfumes or fragrance products together to create a customized effect. While often associated with consumer experimentation, layering can also be a deliberate design strategy.

Designing perfumes that layer well requires restraint and modular thinking. Simpler structures with clear identities integrate more easily than complex, highly specific blends. A soft, woody base perfume, for example, may serve as a foundation for multiple-layered expressions.

Layering highlights the importance of compatibility. Materials that dominate in isolation may overwhelm when combined. Testing layered applications helps identify which perfumes complement one another.

Seasonal and Situational Design

Perfume format and structure often change with season and context. Warmer temperatures increase diffusion and volatility, while cooler temperatures slow evaporation. A fragrance that feels balanced in winter may feel overpowering in summer.

Designing seasonally appropriate perfumes involves adjusting concentration, weight, and format. Lighter formats and fresher structures suit warm weather, while richer bases and higher concentrations perform better in cooler conditions.

Situational design also considers the environment. A perfume intended for close–contact settings benefits from subtle diffusion, while one designed for open spaces may support greater projection.

Adapting a Formula Across Formats

A single aromatic composition may be adapted into multiple formats, but this could mean adjustments are necessary. Each format emphasizes different aspects of the perfume.

Adapting successfully involves identifying the core of the fragrance—the heart accord or defining structure—and adjusting supporting elements accordingly. Top notes may need reinforcement in oil formats, while bases may require reduction in alcohol sprays.

Testing each adaptation independently ensures the fragrance remains balanced and expressive across formats.

Format as an Extension of Design

Perfume format is not merely a delivery system; it is an extension of the design itself. A well–chosen format enhances the fragrance's intention, supporting how it is meant to be experienced.

When structure, composition, and format align, the result is a perfume that feels complete, purposeful, and wearable. Understanding these relationships allows the perfumer to move confidently from formulation to finished product without compromising artistic integrity.

CHAPTER 20

Perfume Creation from Start to Finish

This chapter brings together everything covered in this book and shows how to apply it in practice. When these steps are followed, the result is a perfume that is balanced, wearable, and cohesive.

The purpose of this chapter is to teach a repeatable method you can use every time you make perfume, regardless of style or format.

Step One: Decide on the Format and Container

Before choosing essential oils, decide how the perfume will be used. The container determines dilution, volatility, and how the fragrance unfolds on the skin.

Common perfume formats include alcohol-based sprays, oil-based roll-ons, solid perfumes, and body or bath oils. Alcohol-based sprays diffuse quickly and highlight top notes. Oil–based roll–ons sit closer to the skin and emphasize heart and base notes. Solid perfumes soften evaporation and develop slowly. Body and bath oils must remain low in concentration and gentle.

This decision determines everything that follows. Selecting oils before choosing the format often leads to imbalance or disappointment.

Step Two: Define the Direction of the Perfume

Next, define the energetic direction of the fragrance. This is where you apply what you learned about fragrance families and style.

Ask how the perfume is intended to present itself in use. Consider its overall character—such as fresh, soft, warm, deep, or grounding—and whether it is designed for daytime wear, evening use, or flexible application across contexts.

Some perfumes emphasize floral or softly resinous structures, while others lean toward aromatic–woody or dry–woody profiles. More balanced compositions combine freshness with restrained depth. Defining this structural direction narrows material selection and helps keep the blend focused.

Step Three: Choose the Fragrance Family or Families

Most perfumes are built around one dominant fragrance family supported by a secondary family. Examples include floral with a woody base, fresh citrus supported by aromatics, or woody with a soft resin heart.

This is where accord knowledge becomes functional. You are choosing structure before choosing individual oils.

Step Four: Decide the Structural Emphasis

Determine where the strength of the perfume will be. Most natural perfumes follow this general structure:

Top notes: 20–30%

Heart notes: 40–50%

Base notes: 20–30%

Oil-based perfumes often emphasize heart and base notes more, while alcohol sprays can support brighter top notes. These ranges are guidelines, not rigid rules, but they provide a reliable starting framework.

Step Five: Build or Select Accords

Build or select an accord for each layer instead of blending oil by oil. Each accord should make sense on its own before being combined.

For example, a floral–woody perfume might use a heart accord of rose, geranium, and ylang ylang; a base accord of cedarwood, sandalwood, and frankincense; and a top accent of bergamot.

Step Six: Build the Perfume in the Correct Order

Perfume is built from the center outward.

Begin with the heart accord, which defines the perfume's identity. Add the base accord to provide support and longevity without overpowering the heart. Shape the top notes last, adding brightness and lift carefully. This order prevents dominance issues and reduces the need for later corrections.

Step Seven: Choose Dilution Based on Format

Dilution is part of design, not an afterthought.

Typical guidelines include 15–20% aromatic materials for alcohol–based sprays, 10–20% for oil–based roll-ons, 5–10% for solid perfumes, and 1–5% for body or bath oils. Stronger is not better;

balance and wearability matter more than intensity. Please refer to APPENDIX A for more information.

Step Eight: Rest and Evaluate

Allow the perfume to rest for at least 24–48 hours before evaluation. Natural perfumes often smell unfinished when freshly blended. Evaluate balance, transitions, comfort, and longevity, and adjust only if necessary, changing one element at a time.

Chapter 21

Common Formulation Problems and Solutions

Every perfumer encounters formulation problems. These challenges are not signs of failure, but signals that the structure, proportions, or interactions within a blend need adjustment. Learning to recognize and resolve common issues is one of the most valuable skills in perfume making. This chapter provides a practical framework for diagnosing problems and correcting them efficiently, without dismantling the entire composition.

Most formulation issues follow recognizable patterns. Once you see them, corrections become systematic instead of experimental.

Flat or One–Dimensional Perfumes

A perfume that smells pleasant but lacks depth or movement is often described as flat. This typically results from excessive overlap within a single aromatic family or insufficient contrast between layers.

When too many materials share similar functions or roles, redundancy occurs. The fragrance may smell harmonious but uninteresting, with little evolution over time.

Correction begins with reduction. Identify materials that duplicate one another's roles and remove or reduce them. Introducing contrast in small amounts—such as a fresh top note in a floral blend or a soft wood in a fresh composition—often restores dimension without altering the core identity.

Overpowering or Heavy Blends

Perfumes that feel oppressive or overwhelming usually contain excessive base materials or dominant constituents. Heavy woods, resins, and balsams can suppress volatility and limit diffusion when used without restraint.

The instinct to fix a weak perfume by adding base notes often creates this problem. Longevity achieved through weight alone results in dullness instead of persistence.

Correction involves reducing the heaviest elements and allowing air into the structure. Improving transitions and balance frequently enhances longevity more effectively than increasing concentration.

Sharp or Harsh Openings

Harsh openings are commonly caused by unbalanced top notes, excessive volatile materials, or certain dominant constituents. The opening may feel piercing, medicinal, or aggressive, even if the drydown is pleasant.

Instead of softening the opening with sweetness, reduction is usually more effective. Lowering the concentration of sharp top notes or dominant materials often resolves the issue. In some cases, introducing a gentle bridging material can smooth the transition into the heart.

Allowing the perfume to rest before making changes is essential, as fresh blends often exaggerate sharpness.

Short–Lived Fragrances

A perfume that fades quickly is often described as lacking longevity, but this problem is frequently structural rather than a matter of strength. Increasing concentration alone rarely solves the issue.

Short–lived perfumes often lack adequate fixation or cohesion between layers. Volatile materials may dissipate before they can be effectively anchored.

Correction focuses on improving structure. Introducing a subtle fixative accord, enhancing base support, or strengthening transitions between layers can significantly extend wear time without heaviness.

Poor Transitions Between Notes

Abrupt transitions between top, heart, and base notes disrupt the perfume's narrative. The fragrance may feel segmented instead of cohesive, with noticeable breaks in development.

This issue often arises when accords are built in isolation without sufficient bridging. Materials that share characteristics across layers help guide the fragrance smoothly from one phase to the next.

Correcting poor transitions involves identifying gaps and introducing or adjusting bridging materials. Often, reducing extremes, not adding new elements, improves flow.

Muddy or Confused Blends

Muddiness occurs when too many materials compete for perception, resulting in a fragrance that lacks clarity. This is often caused by overblending or by combining materials with conflicting directions.

Diagnosis begins with simplification. Removing one or two non-essential materials can dramatically clarify the composition. Focus on reinforcing the primary accord rather than supporting every note equally.

Clarity emerges when each material serves a defined function.

Imbalance Between Strength and Wearability

A perfume may be strong but uncomfortable to wear, or subtle but unsatisfying. This imbalance often results from an excessive emphasis on projection without regard for its weight and diffusion.

Strength does not equal quality. A well-designed perfume can be subtle yet expressive, or powerful yet refined.

Correction involves reassessing proportions instead of increasing overall concentration. Adjusting how materials interact often resolves wearability issues more effectively than dilution alone.

When to Abandon a Formula

Not every perfume can or should be salvaged. If a formulation consistently fails to align with its intended direction despite multiple thoughtful adjustments, it may be more productive to set it aside.

Unsuccessful blends still provide valuable information. Documenting what did not work helps prevent repetition of the same issues and informs future designs.

Abandoning a formula is not wasted effort—it is part of the learning process.

Troubleshooting as a Skill

Troubleshooting is not instinctive; it is learned. With experience, patterns become recognizable, and corrections become more efficient. Over time, the need for drastic changes decreases as formulation decisions become more intentional from the outset.

The ability to diagnose and resolve problems distinguishes skilled perfumers from beginners. It transforms perfume making from trial–and–error into a disciplined craft.

Functional Performance Diagnostic Checklist

When a perfume does not behave as expected, the issue is most often structural, not material–specific. Before making adjustments, evaluate the fragrance using the following diagnostic questions. These are intended to clarify *where* the imbalance occurs, not to prescribe immediate solutions.

Structural Balance

- Does the fragrance feel weighted throughout its lifespan, or does one phase dominate?
- Are transitions between the opening, heart, and drydown clear, or do they feel abrupt or blurred?

Behavior Over Time

- Does the perfume unfold and resolve in the manner originally intended?

- Does it maintain coherence, or does it collapse into a single impression?

Context and Use

- Is the diffusion appropriate to how and where the fragrance is worn?
- Does it remain comfortable during repeated or extended wear?

Clarity and Focus

- Does the fragrance communicate a clear sensory direction?
- Are there materials competing for attention, or do they support a unified structure?

Completion Assessment

- Is there a clear structural issue to correct, or is adjustment becoming speculative?
- Would subtraction clarify the composition more effectively than addition?

If a fragrance consistently performs well across these criteria, further adjustment may be unnecessary. When issues persist, identifying the specific category of imbalance allows for targeted refinement, not broad reformulation.

CHAPTER 22

Essential Oil Roles in Perfume Structure

As perfumery skills advance, the ability to select materials by function rather than by name becomes increasingly important. Instead of asking which oils smell good together, the perfumer begins to question what role a material needs to play within the structure of a fragrance. This chapter organizes essential oils by their primary functional contribution to perfume design.

While many oils serve multiple functions, understanding their dominant role provides clarity and efficiency in formulation. These categories are not rigid classifications, but practical guides that support intentional blending.

Top–Note Oils: Lift, Brightness, and Introduction

Top–note oils create the first impression of a perfume. They are volatile, immediately perceptible, and short–lived. Their role is to attract attention, introduce the fragrance theme, and guide the transition into the heart.

Common top–note oils include citrus peels such as bergamot, lemon, sweet orange, grapefruit, lime, and mandarin, as well as light aromatic materials like basil, eucalyptus (in trace), rosemary, and petitgrain. These oils contribute freshness and clarity, but require structural support to prevent rapid fade.

Top notes should be used with restraint. Excessive reliance on volatile materials can result in harsh openings or fragrances that collapse quickly.

Heart–Note Oils: Identity and Continuity

Heart–note oils form the emotional core of a perfume. They emerge after the top notes fade and remain perceptible for several hours. This layer defines the fragrance's character and theme.

Floral oils such as rose, jasmine, ylang ylang, geranium, neroli, and chamomile commonly occupy the heart, along with aromatic herbs and soft spices. Heart notes must balance presence with flexibility, supporting both top and base without dominating either.

When heart notes lack clarity, the entire perfume suffers. Careful proportioning and contrast within this layer are essential for stability.

Base–Note Oils: Depth, Fixation, and Longevity

Base–note oils provide structure and persistence. They evaporate slowly and anchor the fragrance, extending wear time and shaping the drydown.

Woods such as sandalwood, cedarwood, vetiver, and patchouli, along with resins like frankincense, myrrh, labdanum, and benzoin, commonly form the base. These materials influence weight and diffusion and must be managed carefully to avoid heaviness.

A successful base supports the fragrance quietly, allowing lighter materials to remain perceptible longer without dominating the composition.

Fixative Materials: Stability Without Weight

Fixatives slow evaporation and stabilize the fragrance structure. While many base–note oils act as fixatives, not all fixatives are heavy.

Soft woods, light resins, and certain balsamic materials provide fixation without excessive density. These materials are especially valuable in natural perfumery, where longevity must be achieved through structure instead of synthetics.

Fixatives should enhance cohesion rather than announce themselves.

Modifiers and Accentuators

Modifiers adjust a perfume's tone, texture, or emphasis. They are often used in small amounts to shape perception without becoming focal points.

Examples include green notes that freshen florals, subtle spices that warm compositions, or gentle aromatics that add complexity. Modifiers are particularly useful during refinement, when small changes produce noticeable effects.

Understanding modifiers allows precise control without destabilizing the structure.

Functional Flexibility and Context

Many essential oils behave differently depending on their proportions and context. Bergamot may act as a top note, a unifying element, or a bridge between layers. Patchouli may feel heavy or smooth, depending on its use.

This flexibility underscores the importance of evaluation and experience. Functional categories provide guidance, but final placement depends on behavior within the blend.

Using Functional Reference in Practice

Selecting oils by function streamlines formulation. When a blend feels flat, the perfumer can ask whether lift, contrast, or depth is missing. When longevity is lacking, fixative support can be adjusted deliberately.

Over time, this functional approach becomes intuitive. Materials are chosen not for novelty, but for purpose, resulting in clearer, more stable perfumes.

Chapter 23
Fragrance Family Structural Accords

Fragrance families provide more than stylistic categories—they function as structural archetypes. Each family reflects a distinct proportional logic, material emphasis, and behavioral pattern over time. Understanding these structural tendencies allows the perfumer to build accords with clarity and coherence.

The following sections outline common structural characteristics within each fragrance family represented in this book. These are not formulas or rigid templates. Instead, they serve as architectural reference points that help guide proportion, material selection, and balance.

Detailed structural charts supporting these families are provided in APPENDIX G.

Aromatic / Woody

Aromatic–woody structures typically balance a fresh or citrus lift with a defined herbal heart and a dry, stable woody base. Lavender, clary sage, or geranium often form the heart framework, while cedarwood, vetiver, and light resins anchor the base.

These compositions rely on clarity in the opening and controlled dryness in the drydown. Excessive base weight can create dullness, while insufficient anchoring leads to volatility imbalance. Stability depends on the measured wood proportion rather than density.

Citrus / Fresh Citrus

Citrus-based families emphasize immediacy and lift. Bright top notes dominate the opening phase, supported by aromatic herbs or light woods to extend presence without compressing freshness.

Because citrus materials evaporate quickly, structural support must remain subtle. Overweighting the base reduces brightness, while insufficient support causes rapid fade. Simplicity often strengthens stability in this family.

Fougère

The fougère structure centers around an aromatic heart—most often lavender—supported by fresh citrus in the opening and grounded by woods, mossy materials, or soft resins in the base.

Continuity through the heart phase defines this family. The heart must remain perceptible beyond the citrus opening, while the base reinforces structure without overpowering the aromatic clarity.

Woody / Spicy

Woody–spicy families combine dry woods with restrained spice and aromatic freshness. Citrus or subtle spice may introduce the composition, transitioning into an herbal or floral heart before settling into a firm woody foundation.

Balance is essential. Excess spice sharpens the profile, while excessive wood flattens nuance. Successful woody–spicy structures maintain clarity and controlled warmth without heaviness.

Leather

Leather structures are built around smoky woods, resins, and dry spices. Birch tar, labdanum, and styrax commonly shape the leather impression, supported by grounding woods.

Because leather materials are dense and slow-moving, proportions must be carefully managed. Excessive weight leads to opacity; insufficient structure weakens depth. Controlled layering produces refinement without harshness.

Fruity / Floral

Fruity–floral structures balance bright fruit notes with a defined floral heart and a soft base. Fruit materials introduce lift and approachability, while rose, jasmine, or similar florals establish identity.

The base should remain supportive instead of dominant. Excess sweetness destabilizes clarity; insufficient support shortens wear. Proportional restraint preserves transparency and elegance.

Green / Herbal

Green families emphasize crisp, leafy freshness supported by restrained florals and dry woods. Galbanum, petitgrain, or violet leaf often defines the opening character.

Green materials can become sharp if unsupported. A moderate woody base stabilizes without muting freshness. Structural control ensures the fragrance remains polished rather than aggressive.

Gourmand

Gourmand structures rely on warm resins, balsams, and edible nuances rather than literal sweetness. Vanilla-like materials, benzoin, and warm spices form the base foundation.

Sweetness must be moderated through florals, aromatics, or woods to avoid density. The heart regulates richness, while the base sustains warmth without cloying heaviness.

Aquatic / Marine

Aquatic structures create a sense of openness through citrus, cool aromatics, and sheer woods. These compositions favor air and diffusion over weight.

Because marine impressions are constructed rather than literal, restraint is critical. Heavy base materials disrupt fluidity. Successful aquatic designs maintain clarity across phases without collapsing into thinness.

Amber (Oriental)

Amber structures emphasize warm resins, spice, and depth. Labdanum, benzoin, and balsamic materials form the foundation, often supported by florals and controlled spice.

Longevity arises from layered warmth rather than mass. Excessive density suppresses evolution, while insufficient anchoring weakens continuity. Balanced amber designs sustain presence without stagnation.

Musky / Skin Scent

Skin-scent structures prioritize softness and integration. Projection is minimized, and heart and base materials overlap to create warmth close to the body.

Florals and gentle woods dominate, supported by subtle resins. Structural transitions remain smooth. Excess brightness disrupts intimacy; insufficient base reduces persistence.

Chypre

Chypre structures rely on contrast between a bright citrus opening and a mossy, patchouli-led base. The floral heart mediates between luminosity and depth.

Balance is critical. The base must be substantial without overwhelming the freshness. Sustained contrast defines the family's elegance and authority.

Floral Bouquet

Floral bouquet structures center on layered florals supported by citrus lift and soft woods. Rose and jasmine often define the heart, while modifiers add dimension.

The base provides continuity without overshadowing the florals. Cohesion arises from proportional harmony rather than complexity. Transparency strengthens elegance.

Using Family Structures as Reference

These family outlines provide structural orientation rather than strict templates. Individual oil quality, concentration, and blending content will always influence the outcome.

When working within a fragrance family, focus on proportional relationships and behavioral pacing. Observe how each phase unfolds and how materials support or destabilize one another.

Over time, structural familiarity replaces dependency on reference. Families become intuitive frameworks rather than imposed categories.

The goal is not replication of a type, but mastery of its architectural logic.

CHAPTER 24
Perfume Recipes by Fragrance Family

This chapter presents a series of structurally organized perfume formulas arranged by fragrance family, each designed to demonstrate a distinct architectural approach to natural perfumery. Rather than serving as a collection of standalone recipes, these formulas function as compositional models that reveal how proportions, phase distributions, and material interactions determine a fragrance's behavior over time. Each perfume is written as a complete 100–part aromatic concentrate and may be adapted into finished formats through controlled dilution. All materials are natural essential oils, absolutes, or resins, composed at an artisan scale while remaining fully scalable.

The purpose of this chapter is analytical rather than prescriptive. The formulas illustrate how different structural philosophies—whether volatility-forward brightness, heart-centered continuity, resin-driven depth, contrast-based tension, or intimacy-focused diffusion—produce distinct olfactory outcomes. The emphasis is not on ingredient-effect claims but on compositional logic: how top, heart, and base proportions influence pacing, diffusion radius, stability, and drydown development. Each recipe represents a deliberate architectural framework that can be examined, deconstructed, and adapted.

As you work with these formulas, pay close attention to phase progression. Observe how brightness integrates into structure, how the heart stabilizes or transforms the opening, and how the base either anchors, compresses, or sustains the composition. Compare the behavior of different proportional models across families. The goal is not replication, but fluency—developing the ability to recognize structural patterns and apply them intentionally in your own original designs.

The following formulas demonstrate contrasting structural strategies across fragrance families. Read them comparatively rather than sequentially. Each represents a distinct proportional philosophy that can be analyzed, adapted, and expanded.

Structural Model Summary

The formulas in this chapter are organized by fragrance family, but they also represent distinct structural models. Each model demonstrates a different proportional philosophy and pacing strategy. Understanding these frameworks allows you to evaluate fragrance behavior beyond materials and toward architectural intention.

Volatility-Forward

Volatility-forward structures prioritize elevated top-note proportions to create immediate lift and brightness. Citrus and highly diffusive materials dominate the opening phase, establishing clarity and forward momentum. The heart stabilizes the transition, while the base remains restrained to preserve freshness. These compositions favor radiance and movement over density and extended base persistence.

Heart-Dominant

Heart-dominant structures center the composition in the middle phase, where identity is sustained rather than fleeting. The heart accord carries the greatest proportional weight, ensuring continuity beyond the opening. Top notes introduce direction, and the base provides support without compression. This model provides cohesion and a steady presence throughout wear.

Base-Led

Base-led compositions rely on elevated base proportions to create depth and longevity. Woods, resins, and fixative materials anchor the design early, slowing evaporation and grounding the fragrance. The opening offers contrast without dominating. This structure favors stability, persistence, and compositional authority.

Compression-Based

Compression-based models concentrate weight in both heart and base, creating contained intensity and controlled diffusion.

Rather than projecting broadly, the fragrance unfolds gradually and remains structurally compact. Depth is achieved through layered materials rather than overt brightness. This approach is often used in leather, amber, and dense woody constructions where restraint and richness must coexist.

Contrast-Based

Contrast-based structures sustain perceptible tension between luminous top notes and a darker foundation. The heart functions as a mediator, preventing collapse while maintaining tonal separation. Freshness and depth remain active simultaneously rather than sequentially. These compositions depend on proportional balance to preserve clarity without sacrificing shadow.

Diffusion-Driven

Diffusion-driven designs prioritize air, transparency, and fluid progression. Proportions are balanced to sustain freshness without heavy anchoring. Cooling aromatics and sheer woods allow the fragrance to remain open and mobile. Longevity arises from moderation rather than density, preserving clarity across phases.

Intimacy-Based

Intimacy-based structures are designed to sit close to the skin with minimal projection. Materials are layered for softness and tonal overlap, allowing heart and base to integrate seamlessly. Transitions are gentle, and the diffusion radius remains intentionally narrow. This model favors subtlety, warmth, and personal presence over broadcast intensity.

Sweetness-Controlled

Sweetness-controlled structures manage balsamic or gourmand materials through proportional restraint. Florals, aromatics, or dry woods regulate density to prevent excess heaviness. Warmth is sustained in the base, while the heart moderates sweetness to preserve refinement. This approach allows richness to remain elegant rather than overwhelming.

Aromatic / Woody

This aromatic–woody composition is designed around fresh herbal clarity supported by structured dry woods. Built within the aromatic–woody family, it emphasizes balance and compositional stability, pairing lavender and green aromatics with bright citrus lift and subtle spice before settling into a restrained resin–wood foundation. The intended effect is alert composure and grounded confidence, making it particularly suited for daytime wear, professional settings, or transitions that require steady presence without excess projection. Inspired by contemporary aromatic–woody structures that combine vibrant openings with controlled, persistent drydowns, the formula prioritizes clarity in the opening, continuity through the heart, and a sustained yet composed woody finish.

Aromatic Heart Accord – 40 drops (40%)

18 drops Lavender fine (18%)

10 drops Geranium (10%)

12 drops Clary sage (12%)

Fresh Citrus Accord – 20 drops (20%)

12 drops Bergamot (12%)

8 drops Grapefruit (8%)

Woody Resin Base Accord – 40 drops (40%)

16 drops Cedarwood atlas (16%)

10 drops Vetiver (10%)

8 drops Frankincense (8%)

6 drops Labdanum (6%)

Total: 100 drops aromatic concentrate

Structural Architecture Analysis for Aromatic / Woody

This Aromatic–Woody composition is built on a symmetrical 40 / 20 / 40 distribution, creating balance between aromatic identity and woody persistence. The citrus top at 20% provides clarity without volatility dominance, allowing the lavender-centered heart to emerge quickly and maintain composure. Because the heart and base are equally weighted at 40% each, the fragrance sustains continuity rather than contrast. The aromatic core stabilizes the structure early, while cedarwood and vetiver anchor the drydown with restrained depth. The result is steady evolution rather than a dramatic shift, supporting the intended experience of grounded confidence and daily versatility. Minor increases in citrus would shorten longevity, while excessive base would compress brightness. The current proportions maintain structural equilibrium.

Citrus / Fresh Citrus

This Citrus composition is structured around volatility and brightness, emphasizing sparkling lift and clean forward momentum. Situated within the fresh citrus family, it is built on a high proportion of radiant citrus materials supported by airy aromatics and a restrained woody base that prevents collapse without darkening the profile. The intention is mental clarity and energetic engagement, making it well-suited to morning use, warm climates, and moments that require lightness and movement. Inspired by luminous citrus structures that favor immediacy over density, the formula highlights clarity in the opening, gentle aromatic stabilization through the heart, and a sheer, polished drydown that remains fresh rather than sharp.

Citrus Top Accord – 45 drops (45%)

18 drops Bergamot FCF (18%)

12 drops Lemon (12%)

10 drops Grapefruit (10%)

5 drops Mandarin (5%)

Fresh Aromatic Heart Accord – 30 drops (30%)

12 drops Lavender fine (12%)

8 drops Rosemary cineole (8%)

6 drops Petitgrain (6%)

4 drops Neroli (4%)

Sheer Woody Base Accord – 25 drops (25%)

10 drops Cedarwood atlas (10%)

7 drops Amyris (7%)

5 drops Vetiver (5%)

3 drops Frankincense (3%)

Total: 100 drops aromatic concentrate

Structural Architecture Analysis for Citrus / Fresh Citrus

This composition is volatility-forward, with a 45/30/25 distribution that prioritizes brightness and lift. The elevated citrus top establishes immediate diffusion and freshness, while the aromatic heart moderates evaporation and prevents abrupt collapse. The restrained 25% woody base provides skeletal support without darkening the profile. Because citrus occupies nearly half the structure, the heart functions primarily as a stabilizer rather than an identity driver. The design intentionally favors openness over longevity, aligning with warm-weather wear. Increasing base weight would reduce clarity, while increasing citrus further would destabilize progression. The proportions preserve brightness while maintaining coherence.

Fougère

This Fougère composition is centered on aromatic continuity and balanced depth. Belonging to the fresh–aromatic family, it builds around lavender as the structural anchor, supported by citrus brightness in the opening and smooth woods and subtle resins in the base. The effect is composed, fresh, and steady confidence, appropriate for daily wear and structured environments where clarity and presence are desired without dramatic projection. Drawing from the classical fougère tradition while maintaining modern restraint, the architecture favors a clear opening, a sustained aromatic heart, and a grounded woody drydown that preserves freshness rather than allowing sharpness or heaviness to dominate.

Fresh Citrus Accord – 25 drops (25%)

12 drops Bergamot FCF (12%)

8 drops Lemon (8%)

5 drops Mandarin (5%)

Aromatic Fougère Heart Accord – 45 drops (45%)

18 drops Lavender fine (18%)

10 drops Geranium (10%)

8 drops Clary sage (8%)

5 drops Rosemary cineole (5%)

4 drops Petitgrain (4%)

Woody Amber Base Accord – 30 drops (30%)

12 drops Cedarwood atlas (12%)

8 drops Vetiver (8%)

5 drops Frankincense (5%)

5 drops Labdanum (5%)

Total: 100 drops aromatic concentrate

Structural Architecture Analysis for Fougère

This Fougère structure is heart-dominant at 45%, ensuring continuity and aromatic stability. The 25% citrus top introduces freshness without overt volatility, while the 30% woody–amber base provides measured depth. Lavender anchors the composition, supported by herbs and restrained spice that sustain identity through the central wear phase. The near-equal weighting of heart and base prevents either brightness or density from dominating prematurely. This proportional balance produces steady confidence rather than contrast-driven drama. Increasing citrus would reduce fougère character; increasing base would darken the profile. The current structure preserves clarity and composure.

Woody / Spicy

This Woody–Spicy composition is designed around structured woods layered with restrained spice and aromatic clarity. Within the woody–spicy family, it opens with controlled citrus brightness and dry spice, then transitions into an aromatic heart and settles into a smooth, confident woody base. The intended experience is composed warmth and steady energy, suitable for professional settings and day–to–evening transitions. Inspired by contemporary woody constructions that balance clarity with depth, the structure emphasizes polish in the opening, continuity through the heart, and a controlled, persistent drydown that conveys warmth without aggression.

Fresh Citrus–Spice Top Accord – 25 drops (25%)

10 drops Bergamot FCF (10%)

6 drops Lemon (6%)

5 drops Pink pepper (5%)

4 drops Coriander seed (4%)

Aromatic Heart Accord – 35 drops (35%)

12 drops Lavender fine (12%)

8 drops Geranium (8%)

7 drops Clary sage (7%)

4 drops Nutmeg (4%)

4 drops Cardamom (4%)

Dry Woody Base Accord – 40 drops (40%)

16 drops Cedarwood atlas (16%)

10 drops Sandalwood (10%)

6 drops Vetiver (6%)

4 drops Frankincense (4%)

4 drops Patchouli (4%)

Total: 100 drops aromatic concentrate

Structural Architecture Analysis for Woody / Spicy

This Woody–Spicy formula is base-led at 40%, supported by a 35% aromatic heart and a restrained 25% citrus–spice opening. The architecture favors persistence and polish rather than projection. Spice is distributed between the top and the heart to avoid a sharp concentration in a single phase, ensuring gradual warmth rather than abrupt heat. Cedarwood and sandalwood create a structural spine, while lavender maintains clarity through transition. Because the base carries the greatest weight, the fragrance develops steadily and remains grounded. Increasing spice would introduce aggression; reducing base would weaken longevity. The proportions sustain structured warmth suitable for professional settings.

Leather

This Leather composition explores depth and contained intensity through smoky woods and resinous warmth. Structured within the leather family, it opens with restrained spice before moving into a defined leather heart supported by birch tar and balsamic resins, ultimately grounding itself in dark woods that sustain presence without heaviness. The intended experience is quiet strength and grounded authority, particularly suited for evening wear and cooler settings. Inspired by refined leather architectures that rely on proportion rather than excess, the formula balances contrast and cohesion to produce a dry, polished leather impression that remains sophisticated rather than sharp.

Smoky–Spice Top Accord – 20 drops (20%)

8 drops Saffron (8%)

6 drops Black pepper (6%)

4 drops Cardamom (4%)

2 drops Thyme (2%)

Leather Heart Accord – 30 drops (30%)

12 drops Birch tar rectified (12%)

8 drops Labdanum (8%)

6 drops Styrax (6%)

4 drops Clary sage (4%)

Dark Woody Resin Base Accord – 50 drops (50%)

18 drops Cedarwood atlas (18%)

10 drops Sandalwood (10%)

8 drops Patchouli (8%)

8 drops Frankincense (8%)

6 drops Vetiver (6%)

Total: 100 drops aromatic concentrate

Structural Architecture Analysis for Leather

This Leather composition is compression-based, with 50% devoted to the woody–resin base. The 20% spice top introduces controlled heat, while the 30% leather heart defines identity without overwhelming projection. Birch tar and labdanum are carefully proportioned to create smokiness and warmth without medicinal sharpness. The elevated base slows structural movement, producing contained intensity rather than brightness. Because density is distributed across the heart and base, the fragrance evolves gradually and remains grounded. Increasing birch tar would compromise refinement, while reducing base weight would diminish containment. The structure sustains depth with restraint.

Fruity / Floral

This fruity–floral composition is designed around brightness and soft diffusion, blending fresh fruit tones with transparent florals and a clean, supportive base. Positioned within the fruity–floral family, it opens with lively citrus and subtle tartness before settling into a layered floral heart anchored by light woods and gentle resins. The intended effect is lightness and approachability, making it well-suited to daytime wear and warm environments. Inspired by modern fruity–floral structures that prioritize clarity over sweetness, the architecture maintains continuity from opening to drydown, ensuring luminosity without fragility.

Fresh Fruit Top Accord – 30 drops (30%)

12 drops Grapefruit (12%)

8 drops Mandarin (8%)

6 drops Bergamot FCF (6%)

4 drops Blackcurrant bud (4%)

Soft Floral Heart Accord – 45 drops (45%)

16 drops Rose absolute (16%)

10 drops Jasmine sambac absolute (10%)

8 drops Ylang ylang extra (8%)

6 drops Violet leaf absolute (6%)

5 drops Geranium (5%)

Clean Soft Base Accord – 25 drops (25%)

10 drops Sandalwood (10%)

7 drops Amyris (7%)

5 drops Benzoin (5%)

3 drops Frankincense (3%)

Total: 100 drops aromatic concentrate

Structural Architecture Analysis for Fruity / Floral

This fruity–floral design is heart-centered at 45%, with 30% fruit top and 25% soft woody base. The elevated floral core prevents the fruit from fading prematurely and maintains continuity through wear. The restrained base prioritizes transparency over compression. Because sweetness is moderated by floral diffusion and subtle woods, the fragrance remains light without fragility. Increasing base weight would reduce luminosity; increasing fruit would shorten structural stability. The proportions create a balance between brightness and softness.

Green / Herbal

This Green / Herbal composition is structured around crisp botanical clarity and restrained depth. Positioned within the green family, it opens with sharp leafy materials and citrus brightness that establish a distinctly verdant identity before transitioning into an elegant floral heart and settling into a dry, mossy–woody base. The intended effect is mental freshness and natural steadiness, appropriate for morning wear, focused tasks, or transitional outdoor settings. Inspired by refined green structures that balance angular brightness with grounded sophistication, the formula emphasizes contrast in the opening, refinement through the heart, and a cool, composed drydown that preserves greenness rather than softening into sweetness.

Green Top Accord – 30 drops (30%)

12 drops Galbanum (12%)

8 drops Petitgrain (8%)

6 drops Bergamot FCF (6%)

4 drops Violet leaf absolute (4%)

Green Floral Heart Accord – 35 drops (35%)

12 drops Iris (orris butter diluted) (12%)

8 drops Rose absolute (8%)

6 drops Geranium (6%)

5 drops Jasmine sambac absolute (5%)

4 drops Clary sage (4%)

Dry Green Woody Base Accord – 35 drops (35%)

14 drops Vetiver (14%)

10 drops Cedarwood atlas (10%)

6 drops Oakmoss absolute (6%)

5 drops Sandalwood (5%)

Total: 100 drops aromatic concentrate

Structural Architecture Analysis for Green / Herbal

This Green composition relies on contrast between a 30% sharp green opening and a balanced 35/35 heart–base foundation. Galbanum and violet leaf establish crisp identity, while iris and rose refine angularity in the heart. The moss–vetiver base sustains greenness without sweetness. Equal heart and base proportions maintain stability while preserving tension between freshness and depth. Increasing green materials would introduce harshness; increasing base density would darken the profile. The current structure sustains polish and clarity.

Gourmand

This Gourmand composition is built around warm edible nuances shaped through structural restraint. Within the gourmand family, it opens with softened citrus and gentle spice before moving into a floral heart layered with subtle roasted facets, ultimately settling into a resinous vanilla–balsam base that sustains warmth without excess sweetness. The intended experience is comfort and quiet indulgence, well-suited to evening wear and cooler environments. Inspired by modern gourmand constructions that favor balance over confectionery density, the architecture maintains depth and continuity while preventing syrupy heaviness, allowing richness to unfold gradually and cohesively.

Sweet Gourmand Top Accord – 20 drops (20%)

8 drops Sweet orange (8%)

6 drops Mandarin (6%)

4 drops Pink pepper (4%)

2 drops Nutmeg (2%)

.Floral Gourmand Heart Accord – 35 drops (35%)

12 drops Jasmine sambac absolute (12%)

8 drops Orange blossom absolute (8%)

6 drops Ylang ylang extra (6%)

5 drops Coffee CO_2 extract (5%)

4 drops Coriander seed (4%)

Warm Gourmand Base Accord – 45 drops (45%)

18 drops Vanilla absolute or oleoresin (18%)

10 drops Benzoin (10%)

7 drops Patchouli (7%)

6 drops Sandalwood (6%)

4 drops Labdanum (4%)

Total: 100 drops aromatic concentrate

Structural Architecture Analysis for Gourmand

This Gourmand formula is base-led at 45%, with warmth structured through resin and vanilla layering. The 35% floral–spice heart moderates sweetness and prevents syrupy density, while the restrained 20% citrus–spice top introduces gentle lift. Because compression occurs through balsamic depth rather than smoke or dryness, the fragrance evolves gradually and envelops rather than projects. Increasing vanilla would reduce diffusion;

reducing heart weight would destabilize balance. The proportions preserve indulgence without excess.

Aquatic / Marine

This Aquatic / Marine composition explores airy freshness through aromatic transparency rather than literal marine notes. Situated within the fresh–aquatic family, it opens with bright citrus and cooling herbal materials that evoke movement and open air before transitioning into an aromatic heart and settling into a restrained woody base. The intended experience is clean openness and cooling calm, making it particularly suitable for warm weather and daytime use. Inspired by contemporary marine structures that rely on diffusion and clarity, the formula sustains freshness through proportion and restraint, preserving fluidity from opening to drydown without introducing heaviness or sharpness.

Fresh Aquatic Top Accord – 35 drops (35%)

14 drops Bergamot FCF (14%)

8 drops Lemon (8%)

6 drops Grapefruit (6%)

4 drops Eucalyptus radiata (4%)

3 drops Spearmint (3%)

Aromatic Marine Heart Accord – 35 drops (35%)

14 drops Lavender fine (14%)

8 drops Rosemary cineole (8%)

6 drops Clary sage (6%)

4 drops Juniper berry (4%)

3 drops Petitgrain (3%)

Sheer Woody Base Accord – 30 drops (30%)

12 drops Cedarwood atlas (12%)

8 drops Vetiver (8%)

6 drops Frankincense (6%)

4 drops Amyris (4%)

Total: 100 drops aromatic concentrate

Structural Architecture Analysis for Aquatic / Marine

This Marine structure balances 35% cooling citrus with a 35% aromatic heart and 30% sheer woody base. The nearly equal top and heart proportions sustain freshness without abrupt evaporation. The restrained base prevents darkening and maintains transparency. Cooling materials are proportioned carefully to avoid medicinal sharpness, allowing openness rather than intensity to define the composition. Increasing eucalyptus or base weight would reduce fluidity. The structure sustains clarity and air.

Amber (Oriental)

This Amber composition is built on layered resins, warm spice, and deep woods, creating sustained warmth and continuity. Belonging to the amber family, it opens with restrained citrus and spice before unfolding into a rich floral–spice heart and settling into a resin-dominant base anchored by labdanum and benzoin. The intended effect is grounded richness and composed presence, particularly appropriate for evening wear and reflective settings. Inspired by classical amber architecture, which emphasizes depth through proportion, the structure favors gradual development and cohesive warmth, allowing the fragrance to envelop rather than project abruptly.

Spiced Top Accord – 20 drops (20%)
8 drops Bergamot FCF (8%)
6 drops Mandarin (6%)
4 drops Coriander seed (4%)
2 drops Clove bud (2%)

Floral–Spice Heart Accord – 35 drops (35%)
12 drops Jasmine sambac absolute (12%)
8 drops Ylang ylang extra (8%)
6 drops Rose absolute (6%)
5 drops Cinnamon leaf (5%)
4 drops Nutmeg (4%)

Amber Resin Base Accord – 45 drops (45%)
18 drops Labdanum (18%)
10 drops Benzoin (10%)
7 drops Patchouli (7%)

6 drops Sandalwood (6%)

4 drops Frankincense (4%)

Total: 100 drops aromatic concentrate

Structural Architecture Analysis for Amber (Oriental)

This Amber design is resin-dominant at 45%, supported by a 35% floral–spice heart and restrained 20% top. Labdanum and benzoin form the structural spine, producing warmth and longevity. The heart ensures a gradual transition into depth rather than abrupt compression. Because the base carries significant weight, the fragrance evolves slowly and sustains presence. Increasing resin density would reduce refinement; reducing base weight would weaken amber identity. The proportions favor warmth and continuity.

Musky / Skin Scent

This musky/skin Scent composition is designed for intimacy and subtle diffusion. Within the soft floral–woody family, it opens gently with restrained brightness before transitioning into a layered floral heart supported by smooth woods and light resins that blend seamlessly with the wearer's natural scent. The intended experience is comfort and closeness, ideal for daily wear and personal settings where projection is secondary to subtle presence. Inspired by minimalist fragrance structures that prioritize texture over contrast, the architecture emphasizes softness, continuity, and quiet warmth, allowing the composition to sit close to the skin rather than radiate outward.

Soft Floral Top Accord – 25 drops (25%)

10 drops Bergamot FCF (10%)

6 drops Rose absolute (6%)

5 drops Pink pepper (5%)

4 drops Neroli (4%)

Musky Floral Heart Accord – 40 drops (40%)

14 drops Rose absolute (14%)

10 drops Orange blossom absolute (10%)

8 drops Jasmine sambac absolute (8%)

4 drops Ylang ylang extra (4%)

4 drops Clary sage (4%)

Soft Musky Base Accord – 35 drops (35%)

12 drops Sandalwood (12%)

8 drops Amyris (8%)

6 drops Benzoin (6%)

5 drops Frankincense (5%)

4 drops Vetiver (4%)

Total: 100 drops aromatic concentrate

Structural Architecture Analysis for Musky

This Skin Scent composition emphasizes intimacy through a 25/40/35 distribution. The soft floral heart anchors identity, while the gentle woody base provides quiet persistence. The restrained top integrates quickly, preventing projection spikes. Because no single phase dominates, the fragrance blends with the wearer rather than hovering above the skin. Increasing citrus or resin would disrupt softness. The structure sustains closeness and subtle warmth.

Chypre

This Chypre composition is built on a structured contrast between luminous citrus and a grounded patchouli–resin base. Positioned within the classical chypre family, it opens with bright citrus clarity, transitions into a refined floral heart, and settles into a deep woody–resin foundation. The intended effect is poised elegance and grounded sophistication, well-suited to professional environments and composed social occasions. Inspired by traditional chypre architectures that balance brightness and shadow, the structure sustains tension and continuity simultaneously, allowing freshness and depth to coexist throughout wear.

Citrus Opening Accord – 30 drops (30%)

12 drops Bergamot FCF (12%)

10 drops Sweet Orange (10%)

8 drops Mandarin (8%)

Floral Heart Accord – 30 drops (30%)

12 drops Rose absolute (12%)

8 drops Jasmine sambac absolute (8%)

6 drops Ylang ylang extra (6%)

4 drops Neroli (4%)

Chypre Base Accord – 40 drops (40%)

18 drops Patchouli (18%)

8 drops Labdanum (8%)

6 drops Vetiver (6%)

4 drops Frankincense (4%)

4 drops Sandalwood (4%)

Total: 100 drops aromatic concentrate

Structural Architecture Analysis for Chypre

This Chypre composition is contrast-driven, with 30% citrus lift balanced against a 40% patchouli–resin base and moderated by a 30% floral heart. The architecture depends on the tension between brightness and shadow rather than compression or harmony. The elevated base ensures longevity, while the balanced top preserves clarity. If citrus were reduced, the contrast would weaken; if the base were increased excessively, elegance would diminish. The proportions sustain poised authority.

Floral Bouquet

This Floral Bouquet composition centers on layered floral harmony supported by balanced diffusion and polished woody depth. Within the floral family, it builds around rose and jasmine as structural anchors, lifted by citrus radiance and grounded with smooth woods and gentle resins. The intended experience is soft elegance and refined presence, adaptable to both daytime and evening settings. Inspired by luminous bouquet structures that emphasize continuity and cohesion, the architecture maintains clarity from opening through drydown, allowing the florals to remain central while the base provides subtle, sustained support.

Floral Heart Accord – 45 drops (45%)

18 drops Rose absolute (18%)

12 drops Jasmine sambac absolute (12%)

8 drops Ylang ylang extra (8%)

7 drops Geranium bourbon (7%)

Citrus Lift Accord – 20 drops (20%)

10 drops Bergamot FCF (10%)

6 drops Mandarin (6%)

4 drops Petitgrain (4%)

Soft Woody Base Accord – 35 drops (35%)

15 drops Sandalwood (15%)

8 drops Amyris (8%)

6 drops Benzoin (6%)

6 drops Frankincense (6%)

Total: 100 drops aromatic concentrate

Structural Architecture Analysis for Floral Bouquet

This Floral Bouquet structure is heart-centered at 45%, supported by a 35% soft woody base and a restrained 20% citrus lift. The elevated floral proportion ensures layered harmony rather than segmented phases. The base provides continuity without compression, allowing florals to remain central throughout wear. Increasing base density would reduce transparency; increasing citrus would disrupt cohesion. The proportions create refined balance and sustained elegance.

How These Formulas Become Finished Products

Each perfume begins with a complete aromatic concentrate totaling 100 parts. This concentrate remains unchanged regardless of the finished product. Different perfume formats are created by diluting the same concentrate into alcohol, oil, or wax, depending on the intended application.

Alcohol–based products emphasize diffusion and projection and are adjusted by concentration to create Extrait de Parfum, Eau de Parfum, Eau de Toilette, Eau de Cologne, or Eau Fraîche. Oil–based products soften evaporation and keep the fragrance closer to the skin. Solid perfumes slow diffusion further by suspending the concentrate in a wax base. Bath and body oils require much lower concentrations to remain appropriate for broader application.

Finished Product Examples (Artisan Scale)

Extrait de Parfum – 1 oz (30 ml)

Use 7.5 ml aromatic concentrate and 22.5 ml perfumer's alcohol (0.76 fl oz). Combine thoroughly in a glass bottle, cap, and allow to rest for 3–4 weeks before use.

Eau de Parfum – 1 oz (30 ml)

Use 6 ml aromatic concentrate and 24 ml perfumer's alcohol (0.81 fl oz). Blend gently, bottle, and allow to rest for 2–4 weeks.

Eau de Toilette – 1 oz (30 ml)

Use 2.5 ml aromatic concentrate and 27.5 ml perfumer's alcohol (0.93 fl oz). Blend, bottle, and rest for 1–2 weeks.

Eau de Cologne / Eau Fraîche – 2 oz (60 ml)

Use 1.5 ml aromatic concentrate and 58.5 ml perfumer's alcohol (1.98 fl oz). For a lighter splash, up to 0.17 fl oz (5 ml) of the alcohol may be replaced with distilled water. Blend gently and allow a short rest before use.

Oil–Based Roll–On Perfume – 10 ml (0.34 fl oz)

Use 1.5 ml aromatic concentrate blended into 8.5 ml jojoba oil (0.29 fl oz).

Oil–Based Perfume (Dab–On) – 30 ml (1 oz)

Use 5 ml aromatic concentrate blended into 25 ml jojoba oil (0.85 fl oz).

Perfumed Body Oil – 60 ml (2 oz)

Use 1.2 ml aromatic concentrate blended into 58.8 ml carrier oil (1.99 fl oz).

Solid Perfume – 30 ml tin (1 oz)

Gently melt 10 ml beeswax pastilles (0.34 fl oz) with 18 ml jojoba oil (0.61 fl oz). Remove from heat and stir in 2 ml aromatic concentrate (0.07 fl oz). Pour into a container and allow to set.

Perfume Balm (Soft Solid) – 30 ml tin (1 oz)

Melt 6 ml beeswax pastilles (0.20 fl oz) with 22 ml jojoba oil (0.74 fl oz). Remove from heat and stir in 1 ml aromatic concentrate (0.03 fl oz). Pour into a container and allow to cool.

Bath Oil – 60 ml (2 oz)

Blend 1.2 ml aromatic concentrate into 58.8 ml carrier oil (1.99 fl oz). Add to bath immediately before use.

Build each accord separately using the specified drops, then combine them to create a complete 100–drop aromatic concentrate. Allow the concentrate to rest for 48–72 hours to integrate the materials fully. Once rested, dilute the concentrate according to the selected product format, bottle the finished perfume, and allow it to mature before use to achieve optimal balance and performance.

APPENDIX A
Product Types & Concentration Reference Table

Product Type	Typical Concentration	Base Used	Application	Performance Notes
Extrait de Parfum	20–30%	Perfumer's alcohol	Spray	Deep, long-lasting, minimal top notes
Eau de Parfum	15–20%	Perfumer's alcohol	Spray	Balanced diffusion and longevity
Eau de Toilette	6–10%	Perfumer's alcohol	Spray	Brighter opening, lighter wear
Eau de Cologne	3–5%	Perfumer's alcohol	Splash/ Spray	Fresh, volatile
Eau Fraîche	1–3%	Alcohol + water	Splash	Very light, refreshing

Product Type	Typical Concentration	Base Used	Application	Performance Notes
Oil-Based Perfume	10–20%	Carrier oil	Roll-on/ Dab	Soft diffusion, close to skin
Solid Perfume	6–10%	Wax + oil	Balm	Slow release
Bath Oil	1–2%	Carrier oil	Bath	Highly diluted for safety
Perfumed Body Oil	5–10%	Carrier oil	Body	Low concentration, broad application
Perfume Balm	3–6%	Soft wax base	Balm	Gentle scent, low projection

Perfume concentration categories describe how a finished aromatic concentrate is expressed at different strengths. The underlying formula remains unchanged; only dilution and perceptual impact vary. Higher concentrations emphasize depth and longevity, while lower concentrations increase volatility and lightness. Water is not typically used in fine fragrance dilution, except in very light hydroalcoholic formats such as eau fraîche.

APPENDIX B
Drops to Percentage Chart

This drop reference is provided to help visualize proportional relationships within a 100–part aromatic concentrate. It is intended for structural planning and educational comparison only. Drop size varies widely depending on material viscosity, dropper type, and temperature, and should not be used for professional formulation or scaling. Once proportions are established, all formulas should be translated to weight using a calibrated scale to ensure accuracy, consistency, and repeatability.

100–Part Aromatic Concentrate (Professional Method)

In professional perfume formulation, a fragrance is first constructed as a complete aromatic concentrate expressed as 100 parts. Each part represents one percent of the total aromatic composition. This method allows the perfumer to focus on structure, proportion, and accord balance independent of dilution or product format.

Designing a formula as a 100-part concentrate ensures clarity, repeatability, and scalability. Once the aromatic structure is complete, the same concentrate can be accurately diluted into different perfume types—such as extrait, eau de parfum, or oil-based formats—without altering the underlying design.

While drops may be used for demonstration or early studies, professional formulations rely on weight-based measurement for precision.

- 1 part = 1%
- 100 parts = finished perfume "aromatic concentrate."

Approximate Drops

This table provides a visual reference for how drop counts roughly correspond to percentage ranges in a 10 ml working volume; drops are inherently variable and are not used for professional formulation.

Drops	Approx. %
20	10%
30	15%
40	20%
50	25%

Note: Drops are approximate; professional formulation uses weight.

APPENDIX C
Perfume Dilution Chart
(Finished Product Formats)

All perfumes begin with a completed 100–drop aromatic concentrate, which is diluted according to the finished product type.

Perfume Type	Aromatic Concentrate	Alcohol / Oil	Optional Distilled Water	Typical Use
Extrait de Parfum	20–30%	70–80% Perfumer's alcohol	–	Maximum intensity, most extended wear
Eau de Parfum	15–20%	80–85% Perfumer's alcohol	–	Strong, well–projecting

Perfume Type	Aromatic Concentrate	Alcohol / Oil	Optional Distilled Water	Typical Use
Eau de Toilette	6–10%	90–94% Perfumer's alcohol	–	Everyday freshness
Eau de Cologne	3–5%	90–95% Perfumer's alcohol	Up to 10%	Light, refreshing
Eau Fraîche	1–3%	85–95% Perfumer's alcohol	Up to 15%	Very light splash
Perfume Oil	10–20%	Carrier oil	–	Intimate skin scent
Body Oil	5–10%	Carrier oil	–	Subtle all-over use
Solid Perfume	5–10%	Wax + oil base	–	Soft, localized scent
Perfume Balm (Soft Solid)	3–6%	Wax + oil base	–	Close-to-skin
Bath Oil	1–2%	Carrier oil	–	Dispersed in the bath

Distilled water is used only to soften very light alcohol–based formats such as Eau de Cologne and Eau Fraiche. It is not used in higher–concentration perfumes or oil–based products.

APPENDIX D
Drops, Milliliters, and Percentage Conversion Chart

In this book, perfume formulas are structured as 100–drop aromatic concentrates, allowing percentages to translate directly across scales and product formats. Drop counts and milliliter references are provided as approximate visual aids to help understand proportions. Professional formulation relies on weight–based measurement to ensure accuracy, consistency, and repeatability.

(Based on a 100–Drop / 5 ml Aromatic Concentrate)

Drops	Milliliters (ml)	Percentage (%)
1 drop	0.05 ml	1%
2 drops	0.10 ml	2%
3 drops	0.15 ml	3%
4 drops	0.20 ml	4%
5 drops	0.25 ml	5%

Drops	Milliliters (ml)	Percentage (%)
10 drops	0.50 ml	10%
15 drops	0.75 ml	15%
20 drops	1.00 ml	20%
25 drops	1.25 ml	25%
30 drops	1.50 ml	30%
35 drops	1.75 ml	35%
40 drops	2.00 ml	40%
45 drops	2.25 ml	45%
50 drops	2.50 ml	50%
60 drops	3.00 ml	60%
70 drops	3.50 ml	70%
80 drops	4.00 ml	80%
90 drops	4.50 ml	90%
100 drops	5.00 ml	100%

APPENDIX E
Aroma Terminology and Olfactory Descriptors

Balsamic

Warm, sweet, resinous, soft aroma; often rich and enveloping.

Olfactive family: Woody–Balsamic / Oriental–Balsamic.

Examples: Sandalwood, Vetiver, Benzoin.

Camphoraceous

Sharp, clean, fresh, medicinal aroma with a cooling effect.

Olfactive family: Aromatic–Camphoraceous.

Examples: Rosemary ct. Camphor, Eucalyptus globulus.

Citrus

Bright, fresh, uplifting, brisk aroma reminiscent of citrus peel.

Olfactive family: Citrus–Fresh.

Examples: Lemon, Lime, Orange, Grapefruit, Bergamot.

Earthy

Deep, heavy aroma reminiscent of damp soil or roots.

Olfactive family: Woody–Earthy.

Examples: Vetiver, Patchouli.

Floral

Aroma characteristic of flowers, ranging from fresh to rich and heady.

Olfactive family: Floral.

Examples: Rose, Jasmine, Ylang Ylang, Neroli.

Herbaceous

Green, pungent, fresh aroma associated with leafy herbs.

Olfactive family: Aromatic–Herbaceous.

Examples: Lavender, Rosemary, Marjoram.

Minty

Cool, sharp, refreshing aroma with a mentholated sensation.

Olfactive family: Aromatic–Fresh.

Examples: Peppermint, Spearmint.

Peppery

Dry, warm, spicy aroma with a sharp or tingling edge.

Olfactive family: Spicy–Aromatic.

Examples: Black Pepper, Elemi.

Piney

Dry, crisp, invigorating aroma reminiscent of pine forests or needles.

Olfactive family: Woody–Aromatic.

Examples: Pine, Cypress, Fir.

Resinous

Deep, rich, smooth aroma derived from tree resins.

Olfactive family: Resinous / Oriental–Resinous.

Examples: Frankincense, Myrrh, Labdanum.

Spicy

Warm, sharp, pungent, or sweet aroma associated with spices.

Olfactive family: Spicy.

Examples: Clove, Ginger, Cinnamon.

Woody

Dry, warm, long–lasting aroma reminiscent of wood or bark.

Olfactive family: Woody.

Examples: Sandalwood, Cedarwood, Opopanax.

APPENDIX F
Classification by Note Chart

Note placement reflects typical perfumery behavior and may shift with concentration, dilution, and structure.

TOP	MIDDLE	BASE
Anise Star	Allspice	Angelica Root
Aniseed	Ambrette Seed (to base)	Amyris
Basil	Bay	Balsam (Peru / Tolu)
Bergamot	Bay Laurel (to base)	Benzoin
Birch (to base)	Balsam Fir	Cedarwood
Blackcurrant Bud (Cassis)	Black Pepper (to base)	Cistus Labdanum
Blood Orange	Blue Tansy	Copaiba Balsam
Cajeput	Cananga	Frankincense
Cedar Leaf	Caraway Seed	Helichrysum / Immortelle (to middle)

Citronella	Cardamom (to top)	Myrrh
Coriander	Carrot Seed	Oakmoss
Eucalyptus	Cassia	Opoponax
Fennel (to middle)	Chamomile	Orris Root / Orris Butter (to middle)
Finger Lime	Cinnamon	Patchouli
Galbanum (to middle)	Clary Sage (to base)	Rosewood (to middle)
Grapefruit	Clove Bud	Sandalwood
Kaffir Lime Leaf (to middle)	Coffee CO_2 (to base)	Seaweed Absolute (to middle)
Lemon	Cumin	Spikenard
Lemon Myrtle	Cypress (to base)	Styrax
Lemongrass (to middle)	Davana (to base)	Tonka Bean Absolute
Lime	Dill	Vanilla
Litsea cubeba / May Chang	Douglas Fir	Vetiver (to middle)
Mandarin	Elemi (to top)	Violet Leaf (to middle)
Orange, Bitter	Fir Needle	
Orange, Sweet	Geranium	
Oregano	Ginger (to top)	

Palo Santo (to middle)	Ginger Lily	
Peppermint (to middle)	Gingergrass	
Petitgrain (to middle)	Ho Wood	
Pink Pepper (to middle)	Hyssop (to top)	
Ravensara (to middle)	Jasmine Absolute	
Sage (to middle)	Juniper Berry (to top)	
Scotch Pine	Lavandin	
Spearmint	Lavender	
Tangerine	Linaloe Berry	
Tea Tree	Marjoram	
Tulsi	Melissa (to top)	
Verbena, Lemon	Mimosa Absolute	
Yuzu	Myrtle (to top)	
	Narcissus Absolute	
	Neroli (to top)	
	Niaouli	
	Nutmeg	
	Orange Blossom Absolute	

	Osmanthus Absolute	
	Palmarosa	
	Parsley	
	Pimento Leaf	
	Pine	
	Plai	
	Ravintsara	
	Rosalina	
	Rose Absolute	
	Rose Geranium	
	Rosemary	
	Saffron (to middle)	
	Spruce	
	Tagetes (to top)	
	Tarragon (to base)	
	Thyme (to top)	
	Tuberose Absolute	
	Yarrow	
	Ylang Ylang	

APPENDIX G
Fragrance Family Structural Reference Chart

The following chart summarizes the typical proportional tendencies, material roles, and structural risks associated with each fragrance family discussed in this book. These ranges are reference guidelines intended to support architectural clarity rather than prescribe fixed formulas.

Fragrance Family	Typical Proportion Range (T/H/B)	Structural Emphasis	Common Top Materials	Common Heart Materials	Common Base Materials	Primary Structural Risk
Aromatic–Woody	20–30 / 35–45 / 30–40	Herbal clarity with dry woody stability	Bergamot, Grapefruit	Lavender, Clary Sage, Geranium	Cedarwood, Vetiver, Frankincense	Over-drying from excessive wood; heart collapse if underweighted
Citrus / Fresh Citrus	35–45 / 25–35 / 20–30	Bright volatility with subtle anchoring	Lemon, Bergamot, Mandarin	Lavender, Rosemary, Petitgrain	Cedarwood, Amyris	Rapid fade if base too light; dullness if base too heavy
Fougère	20–30 / 40–50 / 25–35	Heart continuity centered on lavender	Bergamot, Lemon	Lavender, Geranium, Clary Sage	Oakmoss, Vetiver, Cedarwood	Citrus dominance; insufficient base grounding
Woody–Spicy	20–30 / 30–40 / 35–45	Dry woods moderated by controlled spice	Bergamot, Lemon, Pink Pepper	Lavender, Nutmeg, Cardamom	Cedarwood, Sandalwood, Patchouli	Harsh spice edge; woody flatness

Fragrance Family	Typical Proportion Range (T/H/B)	Structural Emphasis	Common Top Materials	Common Heart Materials	Common Base Materials	Primary Structural Risk
Leather	15–25 / 25–35 / 40–55	Smoky depth with resinous compression	Saffron, Black Pepper	Birch Tar, Labdanum, Styrax	Cedarwood, Patchouli, Vetiver	Opacity from excess resin; harsh smokiness
Fruity–Floral	25–35 / 40–50 / 20–30	Floral identity lifted by fruit	Grapefruit, Mandarin	Rose, Jasmine, Ylang Ylang	Sandalwood, Benzoin	Over-sweetness; weak base persistence
Green / Herbal	25–35 / 30–40 / 30–35	Crisp green opening with dry woody restraint	Galbanum, Petitgrain	Iris, Geranium, Clary Sage	Vetiver, Oakmoss, Cedarwood	Sharpness; insufficient grounding
Gourmand	15–25 / 30–40 / 40–50	Warm resinous sweetness moderated by heart	Sweet Orange, Nutmeg	Jasmine, Coffee CO_2	Vanilla, Benzoin, Patchouli	Cloying density; suppressed evolution
Aquatic / Marine	30–40 / 30–40 / 25–30	Airy diffusion with light woody support	Bergamot, Lemon, Eucalyptus	Lavender, Rosemary	Cedarwood, Amyris, Frankincense	Thinness; instability from a weak base

Fragrance Family	Typical Proportion Range (T/H/B)	Structural Emphasis	Common Top Materials	Common Heart Materials	Common Base Materials	Primary Structural Risk
Amber (Oriental)	15–25 / 30–40 / 40–50	Resin warmth with sustained depth	Bergamot, Mandarin	Jasmine, Ylang Ylang, Spice	Labdanum, Benzoin, Sandalwood	Over-compression; sweetness dominance
Musky / Skin Scent	20–30 / 35–45 / 30–40	Soft heart–base overlap with low projection	Bergamot, Neroli	Rose, Orange Blossom	Sandalwood, Benzoin, Amyris	Fragility; disruption from excess brightness
Chypre	25–35 / 25–35 / 35–45	Citrus contrast against mossy base	Bergamot, Orange	Rose, Jasmine	Patchouli, Oakmoss, Labdanum	Base heaviness; loss of brightness contrast
Floral Bouquet	20–30 / 45–55 / 20–30	Layered floral heart with gentle support	Bergamot, Mandarin	Rose, Jasmine, Geranium	Sandalwood, Benzoin	Floral muddiness; insufficient lift

APPENDIX H
Material Behavior Reference Table

This reference organizes natural materials by functional behavior within perfume structure. These roles are not fixed note classifications; they describe how materials behave proportionally and structurally within a composition.

Structural Role	Functional Purpose	Common Natural Materials	Proportional Tendency	Primary Structural Risk
Volatile Lift Materials	Create immediacy, brightness, directional opening	Bergamot, Lemon, Grapefruit, Mandarin, Petitgrain	15–40% depending on family	Rapid evaporation; instability if unsupported
Heart Continuity Materials	Sustain identity beyond opening; bridge phases	Lavender, Geranium, Rose, Jasmine, Clary Sage, Ylang Ylang	30–50% in heart-dominant structures	Flattening if under-weighted; muddiness if over-layered

Structural Role	Functional Purpose	Common Natural Materials	Proportional Tendency	Primary Structural Risk
Base Anchors	Provide depth, longevity, structural stability	Cedarwood, Vetiver, Sandalwood, Patchouli	30–50% in base-led designs	Compression; heaviness; loss of diffusion
Fixative Resins	Slow evaporation; integrate transitions	Labdanum, Benzoin, Frankincense, Myrrh, Cistus	5–20% within base phase	Opacity; suppressed evolution
Diffusion Modifiers	Increase airiness or spatial movement	Rosemary, Eucalyptus radiata, Spearmint, Juniper berry	5–15% within top/heart	Sharpness; medicinal edge
Sweetness Regulators	Balance balsamic or gourmand warmth	Clary Sage, Cardamom, Coriander, Light Woods	5–15% within heart/base	Cloying density if mismanaged
Dryness Modulators	Counter sweetness; add refinement	Vetiver, Cedarwood, Oakmoss	5–25% depending on structure	Excess austerity; loss of warmth

Structural Role	Functional Purpose	Common Natural Materials	Proportional Tendency	Primary Structural Risk
Floral Body Builders	Provide fullness and tonal cohesion	Rose Absolute, Jasmine Absolute, Ylang Ylang	20–45% in floral structures	Over-sweetness; diffusion collapse
Green Sharpness Materials	Add crispness, tension, brightness	Galbanum, Violet Leaf, Basil	5–20%	Aggressive opening; imbalance
Structural Bridges	Smooth transitions between phases	Amyris, Sandalwood, Frankincense	5–20%	Blurring contrast if overused
Intimacy Builders	Reduce projection; enhance skin integration	Sandalwood, Benzoin, Ambrette (natural), Soft Florals	20–40% in skin-scent models	Fragility; insufficient lift
Contrast Materials	Create tension between brightness and depth	Bergamot + Patchouli; Citrus + Moss	Variable	Phase collapse if an imbalance occurs

Using Material Behavior Reference Table

1. Identify the family structure you are building.

2. Determine which structural behaviors must dominate.

3. Select materials based on functional role rather than note label.

4. Adjust proportion before introducing additional materials.

5. Evaluate phase behavior over time, not immediately.

Structural fluency develops when materials are understood by behavior, not by category alone.

APPENDIX I
Horizontal and Vertical Accord Reference Table

Horizontal and vertical accords describe two different structural strategies in perfume construction. Horizontal accords enrich a single aromatic layer, while vertical accords establish movement across time.

Accord Type	Structural Focus	Layer Structure	Functional Purpose	Common Application	Primary Risk
Horizontal Accord	Depth within one phase	Top / Top / Top OR Heart / Heart / Heart OR Base / Base / Base	Build tonal richness before full integration	Developing a floral heart, woody base, or citrus opening	Muddiness from too many similar materials
Vertical Accord	Movement across phases	Top / Heart / Base	Create a full structural architecture	Building a complete perfume structure	Imbalance between phases; collapse of transitions

Structural Clarification

Horizontal accords increase density within a layer without establishing full evolution.

Vertical accords create progression, contrast, and time-based development.

Both rely on proportional discipline rather than accumulation.